LUNCH AT THE SHOP

To Anne,
and to lunch!
bon appetit
Peter M
2014

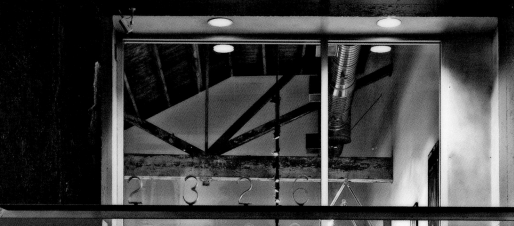
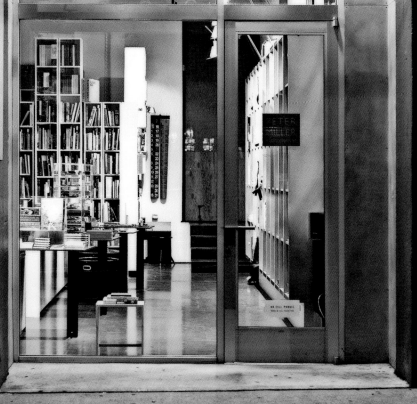

LUNCH AT THE SHOP

The Art and Practice of the Midday Meal

———————

PETER MILLER

With More Than 50 Recipes

PHOTOGRAPHS BY
Christopher Hirsheimer and Melissa Hamilton
DRAWINGS BY Colleen Miller

ABRAMS IMAGE | NEW YORK

Contents

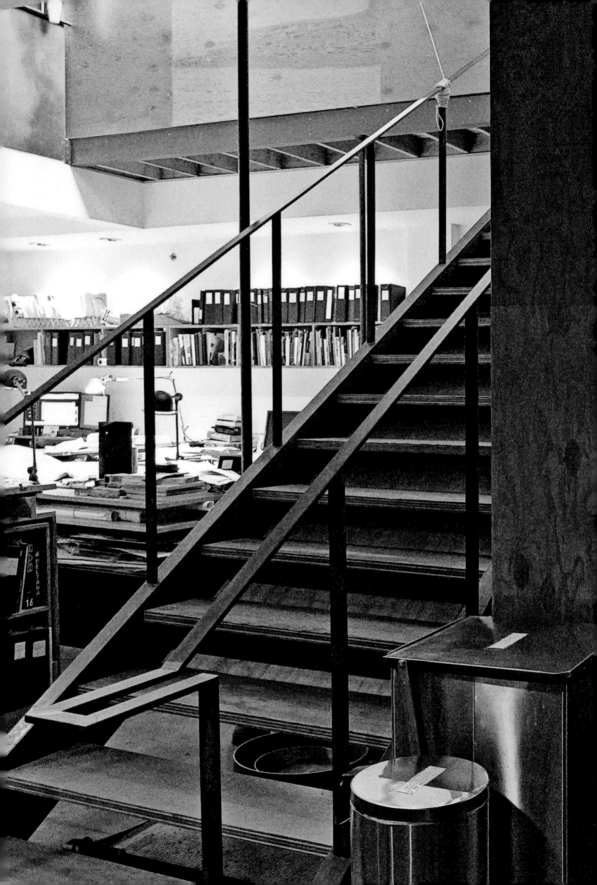

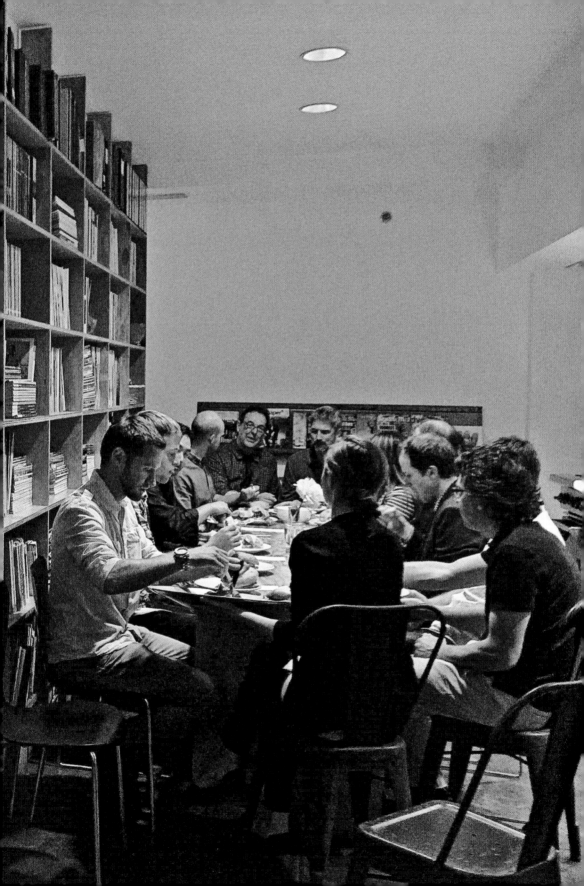

Some of cooking is using food you love.
And some of cooking is using food you have left.
Lunch is about both.

In our current bustle, lunch has been overlooked. The bulk of lunch has been sourced out to stand-up counters and takeout platters, wrapped and rolled and packaged, and it is now mostly a pass-through, of time and of food. We fly on by lunch, as we often fly on by seasons and needs and signals. We have ways to keep us from noting that we are hungry, or tired, or simply need to take a break.

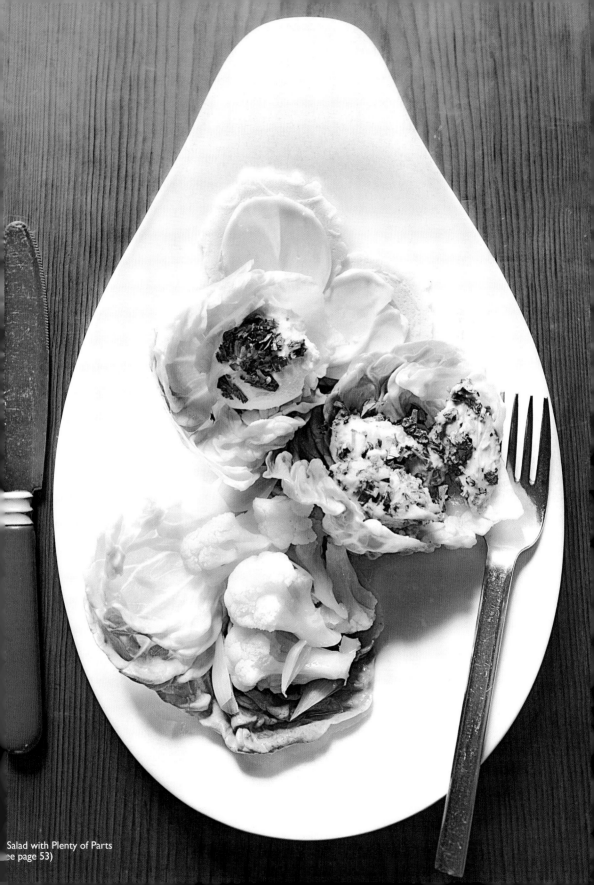

Salad with Plenty of Parts
(ee page 53)

I own a bookshop near the Pike Place Market in Seattle, and my staff and I make lunch every day at the shop, in every season, in all weather, no matter the work that needs to be done that day, adjusting as some things come into market or if some things seem better suited to the mood of the shop. We do not have a formal kitchen—we have neither oven nor cooktop. There are numerous fine restaurants nearby, and a public market, and a park, but most days we prepare and eat lunch in the back room.

It is a lunch made for two, three, or four people, unless others have called in to say they are coming to visit. It is not elaborate—it can be somewhat intricate, but it is more important that it be constant than that it be complicated.

And lunch *is* important. It is, in a way, the good part. It is the separation between the front of the day and the back, a narrow strip between stretches of work. Talking and sitting with others allow us to leave the pencil, or the laptop, or the phone and enjoy the break. We can get back to the work in a few minutes, revived.

It has made a fine difference, here at the shop, and no one doubts that it has changed all of us, improved our workday, and brought us closer together. When people come back to visit, they always visit at lunchtime.

Now that we make it each day, we anticipate it, we sit for it, and, in quiet, subtle ways, we work at it. It can save a workday all on its own, this moment of a little care and community. It is a time to relax and enjoy—no small matter in the gears of a workday.

This book is a manifest to lunch, a script to making a meal for yourself and a few others. It is a call to action, to you, and the people you work with, to share and make lunch together. The job is not complex, and it is not clever. You are simply taking a part of the day back into your own hands, making it personal and a pleasure. The food will be better, the stories more interesting, and the day considerably more distinct.

What Is for Lunch?
We are not always certain what we will have for lunch—but we are always certain it will be fresh and that it will be specific to each of us. We have a kit of things on hand—parsley and lemons, fruit and cheese, pickles and olives, and such—to dress up any meal and make it special. And we always have some combination of beans or rice, pasta or lentils on hand, as well, cooked and ready to go. They are involved, one way or another, in nearly all of our lunches, sometimes as an accessory and sometimes as the main course. They are the proud and historic opposite of fast food.

It is the nature of any lunch at the shop that it be healthy. We select each part of the meal with precision. We are all going back to work, so we make sure to keep the meal from being too hefty or awkward to eat. It must rejuvenate and refuel—it must have some sense to it, a sense of proportion and digestion. There are few sauces to distract or overload, greens are not sprayed for freshness, and nothing is melted on top. The lunch sits out in the open—it has been ready for no more than ten minutes. It was not made to wait in a display case for the day, nor to stay warm for hours.

We keep a sharp eye on the seasons, the local products, and the humor of the shop when sourcing our ingredients—a good lunch will signal what the day is like, both inside and outside. And, of course, it must have a wonderful taste. We have only

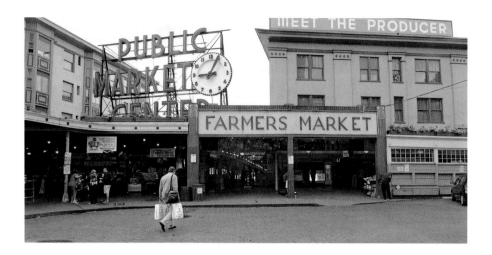

a makeshift kitchen, but it is more than enough for the task. We can dress up and present the foods so they will sparkle and be best of class. A good lunch is not about quantity or labor-intensive preparation; it is made notable by the taste and quality of the food, its thoughtful presentation, and the company it keeps.

Our First Lunch at the Shop

The bookshop opened twenty-five years ago, but we did not always make a lunch there. It started during an annual sale season, when we simply did not have the time to get away for lunch, and we could not think of anything we wanted to order.

I stopped at Frank's Produce and got a head of Bibb lettuce, an avocado, a lemon, a handful of mixed greens, a tomato, and a pear. It was an oddly tentative purchase. "Whatcha makin'?" they asked, and I told them simply, "Lunch." They threw in a small bundle of chives. It was early spring, and the herbs were just coming to market.

Back at the shop, we washed the greens in the big industrial sink out by the freight elevator, delicately shook them dry, and rolled them lightly in paper towels. There were a few plates in the back room and some silverware, but nothing to make a salad dressing.

A fine Italian market, DeLaurenti, is nearby—we went over and got a small bottle of olive oil, a dressy bottle of red wine vinegar, a picnic set of salt and pepper shakers, and a loaf of Ciro's bread. When faced with a ten-foot-long lighted display case of cheese, we couldn't resist ordering a little bit of feta and a tiny chunk of Gruyère. We picked up a bag of Italian cookies near the checkout stand. And I remember thinking, *I wonder if they would cut you eight or ten slices of some of the meats. That would be a lunch all on its own one day.*

We had nothing to make the salad in, so I went over to a nearby bar, the Virginia Inn, and borrowed a very battered stainless-steel mixing bowl. I made a dressing in the bottom of the bowl first, adding some vinegar and salt, then stirring in some olive oil with a fork and some cracked pepper. I carefully unwrapped the lettuce leaves and laid

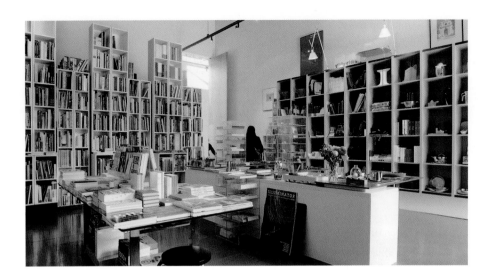

them on top of the dressing, and even more carefully turned them over in the bowl a couple of times to let them all touch the dressing. They fit on the three plates that we had managed to wrangle for the task. There was no place to crumble the feta cheese, so I broke it apart in the bowl and spooned it over the lettuce.

With our single serrated dinner knife, I cut the bright red tomato into pieces, put them into the bowl to sop up whatever was left of the dressing, and then plopped them into the middle of each salad plate. Next I peeled and sliced the avocado, squeezed some lemon on the slices so they would not brown, laid them around the greens, and then squeezed lemon over the top of each plate for good measure.

I had forgotten about the chives—at the last minute, I trimmed their ends and laid three or four over each salad like pick-up sticks. They looked terrific. The pear, cookies, and Gruyère went onto the very last plate that we had, and the bread, torn into sections, went onto some printer paper. Lunch was ready.

We had spent the entire morning talking with customers, helping with sales, checking inventories—but for this moment, there were no customers, no phone calls. We laughed and ate and told stories. And we knew that whatever the rest of the world was having for lunch, no one was having a fresher salad, nor a more welcome break.

That was seven years ago—we have further developed and streamlined the process since then. We now have our own battered stainless-steel bowl, as well as an array of very basic equipment. Our lunches can dress in multiple outfits. We have subtle ways to keep our attention, to pique our interest.

Today our lunches draw from a wider net. We have gotten better at bringing more details into the possibilities of what to serve. For example, we know the best hummus in Seattle is made at Mamnoon, the Lebanese/Syrian restaurant on Capitol Hill. We do not have time to make a special trip there during the workday, but if anyone happens to be traveling near Mamnoon, they know to pick up some hummus, and then we make a meal around it!

The bookshop has evolved, as well. In addition to the five thousand volumes of design books, it now has a kitchen hardware section, with a few elegant pots and pans and lovely dishes. We have used our lunches as a mini laboratory, testing pasta bowls, cheese graters, and water tumblers. Curiously, even though we have access to some of the best-designed products of the twenty-first century, lunch has stayed, deep in its heart, a humble task.

We are the most difficult of critics, being our own customers. Over the years, we have developed an inventory of trusty recipes, ingredients, and techniques, and we are always looking for new and interesting methods of getting the lunch to the table. But the lunch has remained true to that first meal: It is still a pleasure and still a treat. The pear, the piece of cheese, and the cookies are always gone by the end.

A Manual of Sorts

Lunch at the Shop offers advice on the process of planning, gathering, and making lunches. The equipment suggested in the pages that follow will help you make your midday meals efficiently, and the ingredients, the recommended items to stock your shop pantry with, will ensure that the meal has the best chance to taste good and be healthy. The recipes are sturdy veterans, having played at many lunches before. They are chosen to work within the limitations of the workplace.

There are plenty of different kinds of recipes here in the book: meals that can be made at an office desk, meals that can be started at home, meals that can be con-structed from items purchased at stores nearby. Some recipes are specific, and some are open-ended, but all of them have been well tested. We also created a two-week menu that will help if you want a specific plan for how to proceed.

The recipes and advice included in the pages to follow are just a beginning. They are an invitation both to create your own lunch recipes and to see food differently, to celebrate it on a daily basis—not just on special occasions or the weekends. *Lunch at the Shop* challenges you to call on all the allies—the seasons, the shops near you, the vegetable stands, the bakery, the farmers' market, even the flower market. They are all part of making a lunch.

Your Tablemates

To make a lunch every day, in all the varying conditions, you will need a little oomph. The oomph may not always come from the same source. Some days, the season and the market and the dinner from the night before will simply lend themselves to making a midday meal. On other days, you will need another person to carry the momentum, someone else to cobble together parts and pieces into a meal. The recipes and the basic process described in the pages to follow can offer inspiration when it is lacking, but you also have each other. Take turns, share, and fill in when the rest of your crew is too busy to wash, chop, mix, and clean. It is a community, this lunch at the shop, a modest and temporary reliance on each other to help and do what needs to be done. Over time, that community will be the best and most reliable oomph of all.

You can begin with a very small number of people—one or two others is a fine start. You are not trying to make a fuss or a feast; you are simply trying to do better than an isolated salad in a clear plastic package or a shrink-wrapped sandwich. You are sharing the time and the simple effort to make a meal and to enjoy it. In terms of economy, of time and material, it is surely better to make a white bean soup for three or four people than for each to make their own. And it is surely better to gather a few people and have a conversation than to stare at a computer screen.

We quickly discovered that some people rarely, if ever, cook. But with a little guidance, they are often thrilled to help make a meal. We always give any new person a tutorial—how to safely chop parsley, how to properly wash the greens, and how to do the dishes without wasting water or soap or time.

Not everyone at work will help in the same way. We have had people who want to contribute only desserts, and others who want only to be on cleanup duty, not yet trusting their cooking skills. But you can easily ask that someone make a green sauce, or bring in ripe peaches, or pick up a seafood salad from the nearby fish market. The very spontaneity of a lunch makes it possible to use all sorts of contributions.

It is an interesting time in the production of food—there are now more independent growers, vendors, and producers, both in and out of the city, than ever before. Everyone at the shop knows to be on the lookout for whatever would be a fine addition to a lunch, and everyone has a sense of participating in the endlessly varied marketplace surrounding us.

Your official work jobs may all be quite different. But for a lunch, you have a single goal—getting the best possible meal onto the table. You are each the customer, and you are each the cook staff. It is not easy to predict who will do what task. The boss at the office may only be good at dishwashing. It is a new order, and it might surprise you, the passions of food and the pleasures of cooking. They care not a bit for titles—they care only for the food.

And just as we are mining each person's particular skills and interests, there are culinary traditions in all of us that influence the meals. We have had a Persian lunch, a Turkish lunch, a Chilean lunch, a Texas lunch, and certainly others. Each time, it was remarkable how some regional detail—an herb, or spice, or grain—made all the difference. And those details were added to our repertoire.

Lunch is meant to be casual and simple; it is spontaneous enough to not be as intimidating as dinner. Each person can show and tell what they know a backroom lunch to be. With time, lunch at the shop becomes a shared history.

Making the Time

I remember the first true coffee shop in Seattle's Pioneer Square and Mario, the wonderful manager there, trying to make sense of people ordering their coffee to go. He had imagined his customers staying for a few minutes to talk about their first dates, brag about their children, or complain about their bosses while sipping coffee from beautiful ceramic cups with saucers. He wanted everyone to stay a little while, as they would in Italy—to his mind, a short break was too important to pass up, and the coffee tasted better. While stopping to sit and have your coffee every day may not be realistic, the idea of taking the time to relax, savor, and commune is not a foolish one.

Lunch at the Shop argues for stopping for a moment and against certain grains of habit, perceived convenience, and low expectations. Making lunch together is a gentle protest to people not speaking or listening or sharing; it is a counter to a body of people bent in isolation over their cell phones.

In actual time spent, making lunch at the shop is a modest expense. You will divide a few labors, often someone must pick up provisions on the way to work, and there may be ten minutes of prepping. But once you have begun the process, lunch seems to find time to create itself. And in a sense, it is pure self-interest—you are simply investing in a better meal.

Rarely does it seem a chore for us, putting it together. We have been at it for seven years, and we are used to it—spoiled, even. But as you are getting up to speed and adopting new habits, simple but specific things will inspire you and encourage you to continue—good bread and cheese, lovely radishes, a handful of cilantro, or a bunch of grapes. They are the sights and the smells and the touch usually so clearly absent from a workplace (and the usual store-bought lunch). The daily celebration of such things is an easy habit to form. The difficult thing would be to stop.

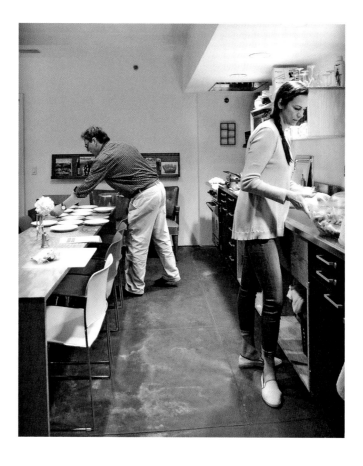

A Few Cooks and the Same Customers

Making lunch at the shop or the office, away from formal kitchens, is a system and a decision. You can rustle up something once or twice; you can haul in a macaroni and cheese from home and say, "Voilà!" But lunch at the shop is a longer prospect than that—it is an everyday affair, through the weeks and through the seasons, when there are no fresh vegetables, when half the crew has a cold, when you have a cold, when no one has a smile or a story to tell. However, with a little help and some company, you can counter even the leanest-spirited days with some fine-spirited meals.

It is a particular pleasure, this process of making lunch in the back. It is a moment's privacy, out of the public eye for a second. It is a moment set aside, away from the computer and the clock. The task itself is a small, specific scenario—leave your workspace, wash up, check ingredients, prepare, and serve—all in ten or fifteen minutes. Roll up your sleeves and make some quick decisions, of a very different sort than the ones that usually dominate your workday: What to add, what to chop, and what would be best for that particular day? It is a craft operation, not a spreadsheet or a program, and it is finished in minutes—completed and reviewed. At its best, lunch is at right angles to the workday. It is a separate stop, not a blur between items on your to-do list.

Making a wonderful sandwich for four people is very different than what most of us do for work. It requires a little caution and a little creativity—the ability to bring together disparate bits and pieces (a bit of cheese left over from yesterday's lunch, the greens straight from the farmer's market, your colleague's favorite salsa). There are colors and textures to fool with, appetites to consider, perhaps a few restrictions of diet, and, always, guests are waiting. Clean plates, napkins, glasses, and silverware . . . lunch is ready.

By taking into your own hands the daily process of food preparation, sitting together, eating, and then cleaning up, you separate the day. By giving lunch some form and detail, you give it grace. By sharing the responsibility, you have the strength of numbers, diversity, and company, as well.

It is a short break. Let the sandwich be the story, or the soup, or the strawberries that have finally arrived. Let the yogurt settle things and the avocado help you recall when it was summer and when it will be warm again. It will, of course, still be nice to go out for a meal. And, realistically, there will be days you have more lunches in mind than lunches in fact. But making lunch at work easily puts you in good company, of both food and people. And it may become a favorite part of your day.

Done well, it has very little cost. Done well, it is fresh and honest and personal. Done well, it will always be a pleasure to eat at the shop.

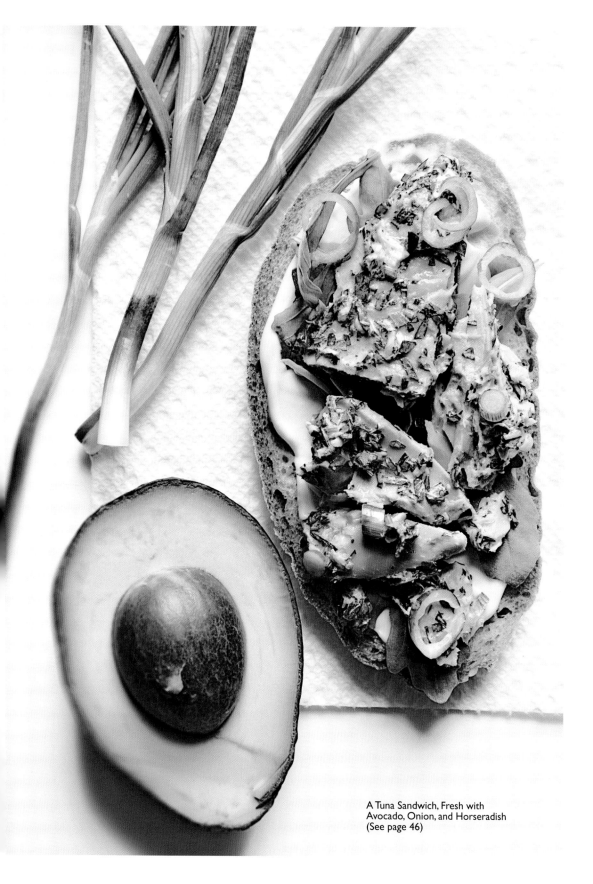

A Tuna Sandwich, Fresh with
Avocado, Onion, and Horseradish
(See page 46)

CHAPTER I
GETTING STARTED:
STOCKING YOUR WORK PANTRY

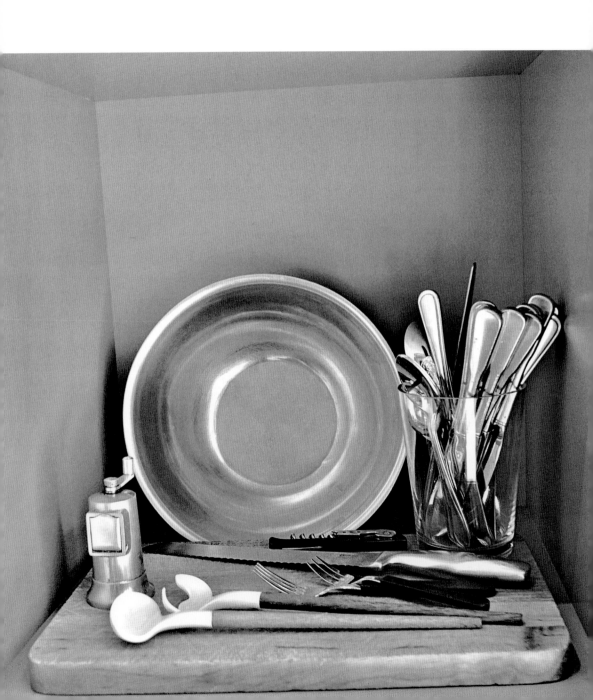

The task of lunch is one of choreography and improvisation. Fewer people or more, less food or more—it is the cobbling together of different foods and different tastes. The right equipment will simplify the work, and keeping a selection of essential food in your larder will give you room to move, adjust, amplify, layer, and garnish. For a good lunch at the shop, we consider all the parts to be essential, with the radish and lemon just as important as the roast beef.

EQUIPMENT:
Bowls, Knives, Cutting Boards, and Such

For nearly seven years, we have made lunch in a limited space with practically no storage, no shelving, and no oven.

There are some pieces of equipment that we consider crucial and fundamental, and there is no idleness to any of them; they must work well, clean easily, and demand little attention. Additionally, they must protect you and protect the food. It is better to have one small good knife than three large clunkers that have never been sharp and that are always threatening to slip off the food. Better to have inexpensive stainless-steel mixing bowls than lovely but heavy ceramic, flower-design bowls, which are liable to slip when washed in the sink with soapy hands. The stainless-steel bowls may get dented like a jalopy, but they clean easily, stack easily, and bounce when they are dropped. Your cutting board should lie flat, and whatever the counter surface, it must not slip or slide. We are making lunch but in very short order and often with a distracted mind—you are at work, after all, and any pre-liminary details that can make your preparations safer and easier should be considered.

Most workplace kitchens are part disaster and part abandon: At one office I visited, the hot-water feed had been disconnected, and that alone had disconnected the people in the office from using the kitchen for anything more than storage. Nothing could be cleaned. There was not a cup or spoon or lonesome fork in any drawer.

The following may seem a daunting list for those facing a reclamation of workspace, but it is, in truth, a list pared to specifics. Much of the equipment can be assembled from extras you have at home or purchased from restaurant-supply stores or even garage sales. Try to gather these few pieces one way or another, for they are essential and will allow you to make lunch in a way that is safe, healthy, and accurate.

Work Area
Claim your territory by cleaning, organizing, and demarcating an area for food preparation. You need to know the counter is clean (and can be cleaned easily), the dishes are not sitting on any debris or below any leak, and the refrigerator and microwave have been cleansed of their past. Food is a lovely discipline.

We purchased a small food-prep table from a supply store, and it made a great difference. No one left his or her coat on it or stacked boxes across it—the quiet authority, perhaps, of olive oil, butter, knives, and a dishtowel.

Two Stainless-Steel Bowls

A small 1-quart bowl and a larger 3-quart version (for making dressings, then for mixing salads, pastas, and such) will be some of the hardest-working tools in your kitchen. If you have the room, you might even consider the extra-large 8- or 10-quart size, which can be a great help with salad preparation. The bigger the bowl, the easier it is to toss the greens in the dressing.

Salad Spinner

Many lunches will involve greens to give the meal life, freshness, and detail. Unfortunately, greens are a Petri dish for cutworms, tiny slugs, and aphids. Even worse, most greens have been touched, sneezed on, sprayed—they have suffered all manners of abuses. You must wash them, and you must be quite rigorous about it, even if their packaging claims prewashing has occurred.

First, you must wash your hands. Then put the greens into a large, deep bowl filled with cool water to soak. Let the greens soak for ten minutes. Local greens can be particularly muddy, especially if there were constant rains where they were grown. You may need to change the water once or twice. Lift the greens out carefully—you do not want the impurities that have fallen off them to grab on again—and place them in the colander insert of the salad spinner. Hold the colander insert over the sink to drain the greens. Shake the colander insert well, put it into the spinner, and spin the greens for a minute or two until dry.

Be careful with the greens, for their sake and for yours. Remember to rinse out the bowl you used for soaking; you are coming back to it with the salad. The salad spinner will require a good rinse each day and will need to be disassembled and given a full soaping once a week.

The spinner is also a lifesaver for fresh herbs—basil, mint, cilantro, parsley, and the like. They are all quick to go limp in hot weather. Soak them in cold water for ten to fifteen minutes and then spin them dry, and they will often be completely revived.

Cutting Board and Breadboard

We use a medium-hard-surface cutting board, 10 by 16 inches, which is large enough to hold a couple of prepped items in a corner while you are chopping another item. Most important, the board must lie flat so that it will not slip while you are cutting. (There are hard-surface cutting boards that clack when you chop on them, and they are helpful for certain work, such as prepping oysters and seafood. But for general lunch tasks, use a softer-surface cutting board, made of polypropylene.)

Use a separate surface for bread, both to protect your knives and to protect yourself. The breadboard may even work best out on the table, away from your usual countertop or work area, giving you more room. If it is a wooden board, protect it by keeping the surface clean and dry. Be very consistent with your cutting boards: By not chopping both vegetables and meats on the breadboard, you avoid having to clean its porous surface with soap and water each time it is used.

A good cutting board will also help the performance of your knives.

Three Knives

A 10-inch straight-edged knife for chopping, a paring knife, and a serrated bread knife (which can also be used to slice tomatoes) will be enough for most lunches. The knives must be kept sharp. A dull knife will be more prone to slipping off the food toward your fingers, making it far more dangerous than a sharp one.

Carrot Peeler, Cheese Grater, Can Opener, and Corkscrew

There are many varieties of each, of course, and most people have two or three varieties in their kitchen drawers. The only important detail is that the peeler must peel and the opener open—basic details but ones not to be taken for granted. (There are more can openers in Zambia that cannot open a can than anywhere else I have ever visited—it is almost a point of honor to wrestle with a can. I brought a new OXO can opener as a gift on my last visit there and made a little speech about its abilities. By the morning, it had disappeared.)

Saltshaker and Pepper Mill

If you can find one, get a pepper mill that can produce both coarse and fine ground pepper. You will appreciate good peppercorns even more when you can vary their effects.

Plates, Cups, Pitcher, Pasta Bowls, Soup Bowls, Knives/Forks/Spoons, Paper Napkins, and Dishtowels

Of the many high-design cooking products that we sell at the shop, only a few have made it to our narrow and particular list of essentials for lunch preparation. Most were simply too fancy for the work. We have only an odd collection of plates and an even odder range of silverware.

We use squat Orskov glasses from Copenhagen. Both oven- and microwave-proof, they hold precisely 1 cup of hot soup, yogurt, or red wine with equal elegance, and they are easily hand-washed. They are an inexpensive luxury and will allow you to serve soup alongside a salad or sandwich without taking up the room required by soup bowls. Because of the clear glass, the soup is visible, which is an advantage over serving it in a coffee mug. (You are not only making lunch, you are making your lunch look better than everyone else's!)

We use a glass pitcher for water. I am always a little surprised by how much water people will drink if it is presented in a good pitcher.

The architect David Chipperfield designed a lovely tableware line for Alessi called Tonale, in several earth-tone colors. We were shipped four Tonale pasta bowls in error a few years ago, and everyone quickly suggested we try them out. They are not inexpensive, but it seemed a worthy experiment. To their true credit, we have never used anything else since then—for pasta or for salad. They have a very helpful shape— flat-surfaced with a 2-inch tapered rim—and they can be stacked. They look wonderful laid out next to each other. The pasta bowls make the meals seem more intimate in scale. Lunch is a daily affair and seems to work best on simple, undecorated plates and bowls.

The shop kitchen has a drawerful of random knives, forks, and spoons for every lunch, and they have never seemed intimidated by the bookshop's display of European flatware. But one piece, a simple butter knife made in Finland for Iittala, somehow made it back into the equipment drawer and has been in daily use ever since.

We use plain white paper napkins for the lunch and dishtowels for cleanup.

Two Rubber Tubs, Wire Dish Rack, Dish Soap, and Sponges

You may not have a dishwasher; we certainly do not. In that case, you will need something in which to hold dirty dishes, wash them, and dry them. A few rubber tubs and a dish rack can be a great help for stacking dirty dishes or letting clean ones dry.

No one likes washing dishes—certainly not at work—so we soften the task by giving it a little attention, using a natural sponge and a dishwashing liquid that is both eco-friendly and sweet smelling. Small matters, surely, but crucial, especially over the course of many lunches. You must keep everything quite clean, or the task itself becomes dreary . . . and unhealthy.

Refrigerator, Microwave, and Panini Press

In any size or shape, they are each important. Since many office kitchens do not have ovens or stoves, none of our recipes call for pots or pans to be used in the shop. If you choose to microwave your food, do so only in glass containers, never plastic.

If you have concerns about using the microwave, you could buy a single-burner gas stove top that can be used inside. Electric cooktops, too, are now quite sophisticated and capable. If you use a cooktop, you will need a good saucepan with a lid and an 8-inch sauté pan.

You could skip the panini press, but it is a great help in reviving stale bread and weary palates. Any soup or salad is quickly lifted by grilled slices of bread that have been rubbed with a little garlic, olive oil, salt, and pepper—or even a bit of basil.

Storage Containers

You can become a crazy person about storage containers. But if you keep your senses, you may come to see that food storage offers, in truth, a particularly insightful look into any culture.

I had always collected matchboxes in my travels, but now, in any new country, I find the kitchen store, the supermarket, or the hardware store and check out the food containers. My daughter looks for the best new versions in Stockholm and gives them to me for the holidays. It is amusing for her to watch me examine each new variety.

The Swedes have their versions, the Finns theirs, and the Danes theirs, as well, all intensely researched and designed to be economical, eco-friendly, aesthetically pleasing, basic, specific, and often brilliant. And this is simply a sampling from Scandinavia.

If you charge your traveling friends with bringing back containers from their journeys, you will get a sense of the wide range of products. But no matter where they are from, food containers must not leak, stain, or grow foul. They must protect, display, endure, and, in some cases, be lovely.

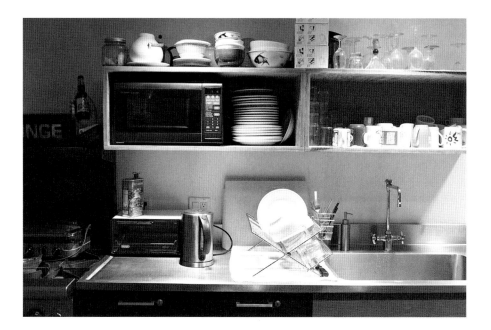

Start with the basics: containers that are both airtight and nontoxic. You will need a few small ones for sauces and a few larger ones for soups and pastas and stews. It is important that you be able to either see or identify what is in them. Be certain which ones are microwavable and which ones are stackable. If you find yourself meeting after work and discussing food containers, however, you have perhaps gone too far down the right track.

Duralex in France makes wonderful glass containers for storage, heating, and serving. Their glasses can also hold hot soups. Bormioli in Italy makes the larger glass storage containers we favor for pastas and meats. Weck, a hundred-year-old German firm, has a handsome glass storage system with very simple clips and rubber seals. And OXO, from New York City, has developed stackable, leak-proof containers that bring order to a fridge. We also keep a selection of reusable empty 32-ounce plastic yogurt containers around for the times when less fancy will work. (These, however, do not go into the microwave.)

At a cooking site, not a full-fledged kitchen, the role of food containers is more crucial and more intricate. Under the best circumstances, newly filled containers will be arriving at the shop as newly cleaned containers are heading out for more supplies.

Setting the Table

We have varied plates and forks and glasses here at the shop, some better than others. But we are very consistent about one thing: We always set the table. We never serve lunch without place mats. They need not be more than the sheets from last year's calendar, the brown wrapping from a package, or the blank back pages from a half-

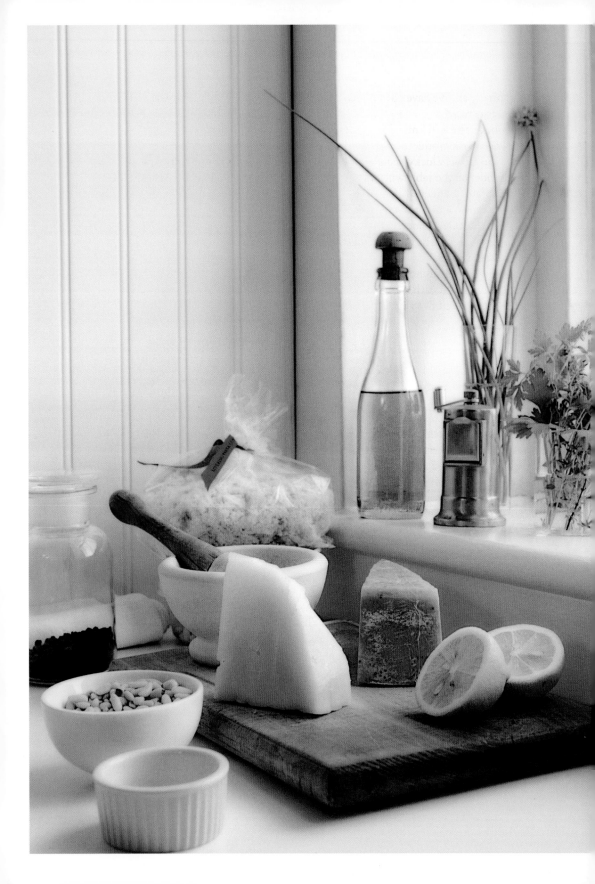

used ledger pad. We have cut out two sides of a shopping bag and made some elegant settings that way.

Fork on the left, knife and spoon atop a napkin on the right—it makes all the difference in the world.

If you are very lucky, then you have a place near your work that sells fresh flowers; having them on the table will add a true touch of elegance to a lunch. You need not buy elaborate bouquets. A few tulips in the spring, a couple of peonies in June, the roses of August, and the summer dahlias—they are the colors of a season. By fall, you can add the lovely geometry of dried flowers and branches to the asters. By winter, you are confined to the colors and flowers of other climates and hemispheres and to dreaming of spring.

Buying flowers is not an easy habit to maintain. I knew a man who wrote into his will that, after his death, a rose should be delivered to his wife every week for the rest of her life. He died five years ago and is still getting credit.

ESSENTIAL FOODS:
Specific On-Site Ingredients

These essential foods are the heart of what you will be making for lunch—if you want to scrimp, try to do it on something else (perhaps fuel consumption). There will be days that are carried and rescued by the quality of these products, days when your spirits have flagged but the essentials bring you back up.

It is not necessary to have all the essentials on hand at the same time. Some essentials, such as breads or meats or cheeses, are conditional. We keep a feta on hand as much as possible, for it can brighten a salad or make a very small amount of lentils seem consequential. If there is a reason to celebrate or luxuriate, be it success or not, we often splurge on prosciutto; it is expensive—in a way, the Champagne of meats. Even one slice, laid on a plate with a little fig paste and a chunk of Parmesan, can, like a glass of bubbly, bring a smile.

The sauces are also conditional. They are very fragile and last only a few days. When you decide to make a green sauce (see page 35), for example, plan to use it all, either at first or over a couple of days. It is wonderful, but you must keep track of it. If you have extra, then adjust the next day's meal into something that also benefits from a green sauce. Nothing can make the task of lunch more burdensome than a refrigerator filled with forgotten food.

Depending on season and taste, some essentials will figure prominently at one time and less at another. We grew accustomed to the pickled onions from the Boat Street Cafe in Seattle, using them to bolster sandwiches and grains or anything that needed propping up. When Boat Street stopped their production for six months, every sandwich seemed to miss that sweet taste. While we never did find a replacement that we liked as much, it gave us a chance to experiment with other pickles, condiments, and garnishes.

Some of the foods are permanent features. We always keep Parmesan on hand, and always the Reggiano brand. It is expensive, but it is the horn section to this orchestra and earns its keep each time we use it. Even the last dried piece can, when grated over a soup or pasta, draw out a freshness and taste that simply do not exist otherwise.

Do not be intimidated by the list of essentials. The most important requirement is that you carefully select everything in your pantry—that you are always conscious of the difference that a good vinegar, for example, will make over a poor one. Lunch is quickness, and a few strokes make all the difference.

PERMANENT FEATURES:

Salt and Pepper
We use a French sea salt with a medium grind—Maldon is one of our favorites, but so is a new salt from Oregon called Jacobsen. We never use flavored salts. And for pepper, we buy Tellicherry berries from the World Spice Merchants just behind Pike Place Market. You will smell their peppercorns immediately when you grind them. They take their products very seriously and can list the dates when the peppercorns were dried. To them, most commercial peppercorns are like a cappuccino made yesterday: flat, stale, and spent.

While the World Spice Merchants might not be at your doorstep, you can still find a local provider of good pepper with a similarly vibrant scent. The world of spices can seem a true demimonde: Wars have been fought and lives lost in the singular pursuit of spices.

Olive Oil
You are not sautéing, which can involve a large quantity of olive oil, so move up a notch and buy a very good brand. You will use it for the dressings and for topping food, and you will taste it directly. In fact, do taste it: If it is terrible or too strong, then choose another. If your vendor won't let you taste it, go somewhere that will. You may want to use a heavier oil in the winter months and a lighter one for summer, adjusting the salt or vinegar you use with each variety. Summer greens, for example, are more tender than well-traveled winter greens, and the olive oil can have a lighter touch.

There are flavored olive oils available, but we avoid them. Good olive oil is its own flavor. Of particular new fame are truffle oils; not only does the smell permeate everything and then die after opening, but it is a contrived and insolent smell. Avoid them all, and, one day, buy a truffle, shave it over hot buttered pasta, and grate some Parmesan cheese onto it—in that moment, you shall taste the brilliance of truffles.

Wine Vinegar
Either red or white wine vinegar will do the trick. Again, you will be tasting it directly in your lunch, so make it an authentic brand. Vinegar and lemon are particularly

important to lunch—they are wonderful revivers and refreshers. Just as they serve to keep food from browning, so do they enliven and lighten it.

Lemon

When I see a lemon on our counter, I know we can make lunch.

Balsamic Vinegar

You could put this aged Italian vinegar on the heel of an old walking shoe and probably still feel a temptation to taste it. It is quite easy to find yourself using balsamic vinegar every day, but that is too often. Balsamic vinegar should be used in drops, not streams—its impact is immediate, so exercise restraint! Use it *beside* instead of *on* the food. There is a great and historical range to this vinegar and a corresponding range to its price. For lunch, you do not need the twenty-five-year-old variety, cave-aged by elders in Modena, but a little bottle of good-quality balsamic should serve you well.

Parmigiano-Reggiano

Try to keep one cheese always on hand: a one-pound slab of Parmesan, and always Parmigiano-Reggiano. You will grate it into soup, over salad, over pasta; you will crumble it as a side dish with apples and pears or shave it on top of a fresh spring salad or the finally fresh summer tomatoes; or you will indulge yourself and serve it in small chunks with honey and a dab of fig paste or pickled plums. It is a true and loyal cheese. And it loves the work. You must experiment with containers for it, as it will dry out with too much air or will strangle if it is sealed in plastic and can get no air at all. We use an old plastic box with a snap lid that seems to breathe just enough to keep the Parmesan stable.

Condiments

You must be careful, especially at work, that you do not overwhelm yourself with condiments. In general, they do keep well, but if the selection gets too broad, they become difficult to manage, to remember, and to find. We keep only a few.

Chutney: There are many varieties, but our choices are mango, green chili, or lemon. In the fall, you can often find a tomato chutney. Chutney is like a brightly colored shirt or scarf—in both taste and color, it helps break up the routine of a lunch. Even a touch at the side of a plate can make a big difference. Try chutney with chicken or beef or next to a rice dish. And keep in mind, chutney has thrived for more than two thousand years by its charm and wit.

Mustard: Find a Dijon that you love, and make certain you always have it on hand. We choose a smooth mustard, not a grainy one, so that it can mix completely in dressings.

Fig spread and French plum spread: You may only use them a couple of times in a month, but they can both bring a sweetness to a dish that, for whatever reason, seems stubbornly dull. Add a teaspoon of the fig when you have good sliced ham, or some of the plum when you serve chicken, or add either of them to a tartine.

Honey: We did not keep any honey on hand at first, but then Jessie, one of the store managers, came back to work after a short sabbatical (she missed the lunches)

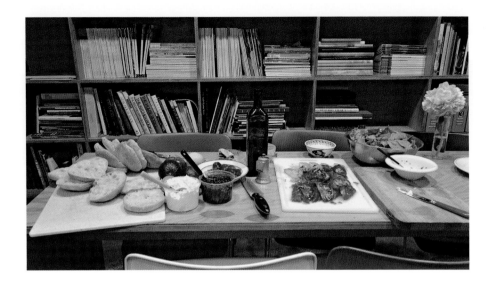

and brought two jars of honey, labeled Gloria and Lorene (after her grandmothers), from her own hive here in Seattle. In a month, they were both empty. It is a wonderful midmorning snack on a single slice of bread or stirred into a couple of tablespoons of yogurt. And it is a brilliant after-lunch dessert for days that might need such a thing. We would simply cut a slice of hard cheese—a Gruyère or, best of all, a young Parmesan—and lay some honey beside it with a couple of slices of pear or a crisp apple. The honey, like the bees, then does all the work.

Accompaniments

Simple sandwiches and salads and soups often need a little something extra to take them to the next level, something crunchy or salty or sweet. We always keep these trusty sidekicks on hand.

Olives: There are thousands of kinds of olives, and they each have seasons in which they thrive and seasons when they can taste old. They are not timeless. We have a couple of guidelines: Always taste the olives first, never buy them without their pits, never buy a mixture of olives, and always store them in their brine. We will often serve them before lunch with a fresh grinding of pepper, some sea salt, a rosemary branch (if we have one), and some good olive oil, for the taste and the color. When you serve them, try to choose a plate or bowl that shows off their color and the color of the oil—it will make a difference.

Marinated onions, or other veggies: There is a wonderful restaurant in Seattle, called the Boat Street Cafe, which serves marinated fruits and vegetables with all of their courses. They now offer some of them in grocery stores. The marinated red onions are our favorite, sweet and sour and spicy, and just the thing for a once-dry sandwich or a still-dull salad. While pickles once seemed old-fashioned, they have been revived and restored for their subtle addition to meals and even subtler economy. Check your food stores and seasonal markets for local brands of pickled onions—or cauliflower, plums, carrots, watermelon, or the like.

CONDITIONAL FEATURES:

Bread

You may need to go out of your way for the best bread, but after a while the trip will not seem out of the way. The bread may be a baguette, a Parisian, a dense loaf, a *pain de campagne*, or a thickened sour rye.

The difficulty is finding truly good bread. There are elaborate ways for any grocery store, large or small, to offer fresh-baked bread or bagels or rolls; this is a clever country, and the vendor can buy the frozen dough for any imaginable concoction. They need only let it rise, toss it into the oven, and set the timer; twenty-eight minutes later, the bell goes off, and you have a loaf. It is a miracle of science and convenience, but the bread winds up somewhat empty of taste.

Be a snob and a realist about bread. If you can get to a baker, then lucky you. There are countless lunches laid on the shoulders of good bread. Open-faced sandwiches, for example, with a bit of butter and a single slice of ham, or a piece of fruit and cheese on top—all are possible only because the bread is so good.

Our nearest bakery makes a dense country white loaf that can be thickly sliced and then grilled and served open-faced with goat cheese, olive oil, chives, basil, or just extra pepper. That alone is nearly lunch enough.

If you cannot access good bread, then you must improvise and be clever. If you want a fine role model, let it be a Vietnamese sandwich, the *bánh mì*. It is a brilliant example of overcoming the plainness of commercial bread with a complexity of sauces, marinades, seasonings, picklings, greens, and bits of meat. It is a colorful parade inside a very plain shell.

Keep an eye out for other alternatives (pitas, tortillas, and flatbreads), for there are often very fresh and handmade versions that remain available only because the neighborhood favors them. These breads are the literal version of what can be done when there is not a proper baking oven, when there is neither time nor source nor climate for bread rising.

Here again is an argument for having a panini press on hand. It will give you some wonderful options in handling bread. Pita can be reheated easily; *bollo* rolls that seem damp or stale can be revived by grilling them with olive oil—or, better yet, lay a slice of Gruyère and dab of mustard in the middle and grill the roll until the cheese melts. And any day-old bread, if sliced and lightly touched with olive oil, can be grilled, salted, and placed below a soup or stew.

Other Cheeses

For cheeses other than our constant friend Parmesan, we have been most successful when we use them right away as a main ingredient in our lunches and focus on using any remaining cheese in subsequent days. If we buy goat cheese, then we use it the

ON BREAD ALONE

For years, there were few artisanal bakeries anywhere in America. I can well remember when Ciro Pasciutto opened his bakery, La Panzanella, here in Seattle in the late 1980s. Ciro is a big man and he liked to bake very large loaves of Italian country white bread, loaves as long as a bed pillow and nearly as wide. He would drive around delivering these monsters before anyone was awake, and each week would leave one propped against our bookshop front door. We would cut it into quarters and even the quarter sizes were a handful. We made sandwiches with it but more often we simply piled slices on a plate and let people dip into olive oil or any sauce such as hummus.

Ciro's bread would stay fresh for a couple of days—then, knowing Ciro would ask, you would carefully convert the leftover bread into stuffing or bread crumbs. It was a code that you must never throw any bread away.

In Belltown, where we have the bookshop, there is a bakery, Macrina, that is so beloved that directions are given and distances calculated in specific relation to the bakery. They make many fine breads—wheat and olive and potato and herb and walnut—but our favorite is a roll, a ciabatta roll. We will order some in advance for our lunches; they only seem to keep three or four of them on hand, not enough for the appetite of our crew. It is the perfect roll. The outside has a slight crust but the interior is soft and modest, ideal for the spinach and ricotta sandwich (see page 48).

As loyal as we are to the ciabatta roll, if we happen to be twenty blocks south, in Pioneer Square, we will always stop at the Grand Central Bakery and pick up two or three semolina baguettes. It is particularly memorable when eaten within four hours of baking with a sweet ham, French mustard, and a sharp cheese.

It is a difficult task, to run a bakery and to make good bread. It involves long and very early hours, a stubborn steadfastness, and always a sense of the air and the weather and the flour and the yeast. When you find a good bakery, you will also have found the inspiration and the starting place for making your own lunches. The bread itself has done its job, setting a pace of care and quality.

first day as a main course, and if there is any left, we finish it as a side dish the second day. Feta is also a wonderful assistant in creating lunch. It can freshen any salad, or any fruit, or any soup. It can be dressed with olive oil touched with mint or cilantro or basil. If you store it in a container with water (adding a little salt to the water), it will often keep for more than a week.

Keep blue cheese in mind as a reserve, like the French horn or, perhaps, cymbals in the orchestra. The most famous—Roquefort, Stilton, Gorgonzola—have many labels and grades and are available in any cheese case. They are true veterans, many of them having been in production for hundreds of years. But now there are also newcomers, local cheese-makers braving the interaction of penicillium and sheep's milk. Look for them at your local farmers' markets. Some are young, some are rough textured, and some are brash and sassy. It's an intriguing cheese type to explore.

Use blue cheese on crackers or thinly sliced dark rye bread, sometimes with a little butter beneath. It is also wonderful when crumbled slightly with a fork and mixed for a moment with cooked beets or tossed into a very green salad. The blue cheese is a sprightly braggart, a wonderful contrast to green leaves and fresh red tomatoes. It loves cracked black pepper or even a drop of vinegar. But to my mind, blue cheese is best used in two very simple ways: completely by itself as a slice or next to a ripe pear or a fresh fig in early fall.

It can be difficult to keep track of different cheeses, so it can be helpful to set a routine. We buy feta, for example, most Monday mornings and try to use all of it (for four people in a week: one pound) by the weekend. The *Fromager d'Affinois* is the key ingredient for our favorite sandwich (see page 44), especially in the fall and winter, so we will buy a half pound every other week. And the blue cheese is a great treat, but we tend to wait for treats—we seem to buy blue cheese once a month, but once a week in October when the pears are perfect and it seems foolish not to end every Friday lunch with pears and a blue.

Yogurt

Yogurt is a fascinating product. Thirty years ago, it seemed to have pigeonholed itself into a faux dessert or shy indulgence. But it escaped such taming, and today it has quietly become a very subtle and brilliant ambassador for the cuisine of many countries. In the gentlest of ways, it has brought the cooking of Greece, Turkey, Egypt, Syria, and Israel into a global vernacular. It has digestive and other general health benefits, speaks hundreds of languages, and is beloved from Nepal to New Jersey. It has made certain spices and herbs—cumin and coriander, cilantro and cayenne—into essentials for soups and salads and sauces. And it has moved sour cream and cottage cheese into quite minor, dour-faced roles.

A Spiced Yogurt

MAKES 1 CUP.

1 cup Greek yogurt

1 teaspoon cumin

2 teaspoons olive oil

Salt

Freshly ground black pepper

Mix the yogurt with the cumin, then the oil. Taste and add the salt and pepper as needed. Lay a spoonful of the spiced yogurt beside any rice or lentil dish. For instance, it would be perfect with the lentil soup on page 74.

Yogurt is a brilliant ally when making lunch, ready at all times to be sweet or sour, set alone, or mixed intimately with other flavors. If you had the chance to visit a supermarket in Paris, you would in a moment realize the cultural glamour of yogurt. There are always hundreds of varieties on display.

Use it as a side dish mixed with a bit of garlic and fresh herbs. Use it as a binder combining lentils and chopped vegetables. It is a wonderful aid to a sullen half-cup of soup and a bright change to the repetition of salad dressings. Try a dollop next to a sliced pear for dessert. There is a freshness to yogurt, and it has a remarkable talent for befriending characters as varied as a spicy, grizzled sausage or a sweet red strawberry.

Herbs

We keep five herbs in rotation—not all of them together and not all of the time—including: parsley, basil, chives, mint, and cilantro. There was a time, perhaps ten years ago, that such a collection would have been considered exotic. But improved packaging and demand have made them easily available.

They often keep for more than a week in the refrigerator, but they demand attention: You must use them and enjoy them, or they will quickly seem a foolish luxury. The packaging for herbs is subtle, allowing some air circulation but retaining some moisture, and that lengthens their shelf life. Keep herbs in their packaging and refrigerate them, adding a few drops of water every other day or so. If you are buying herbs from a

CILANTRO AT THE SHOP

We did not use cilantro often at lunch until we received some visitors from the School of Architecture in Mexico City. Four professors and sixteen students were in Seattle for a week, and they taught all of us much wider dimensions of work hard/play hard. They loved to eat and to work and to cook and to laugh and to look at books. I was making a lunch and invited some of them to join us.

There I was, chopping this scrawny stem of cilantro to add to the avocado. Javier Sanchez, an award-winning architect and one of the school's most celebrated professors, laughed and said he would help. He came back from the market with an armload of cilantro and avocados and limes, more of each than I would use in two months. He chopped and scooped and squeezed and told stories and produced the most luscious guacamole and the freshest salmon tartar we had ever tasted. And that may be the key to cilantro—use it with exuberance. It is a cutter, a kind of thin, green blade within the tastes of other staples.

It was fascinating how easily the students understood the nature of a lunch at the shop, though they had never been to our shop before. Sent out to gather ingredients so we could all eat together, they scattered in small groups and returned with just the right items: fruits to be sectioned, fresh cheeses, salsa, long, skinny loaves of bread, roasted almonds, and a ceviche from the Japanese fishmonger. A lunch was ready in moments.

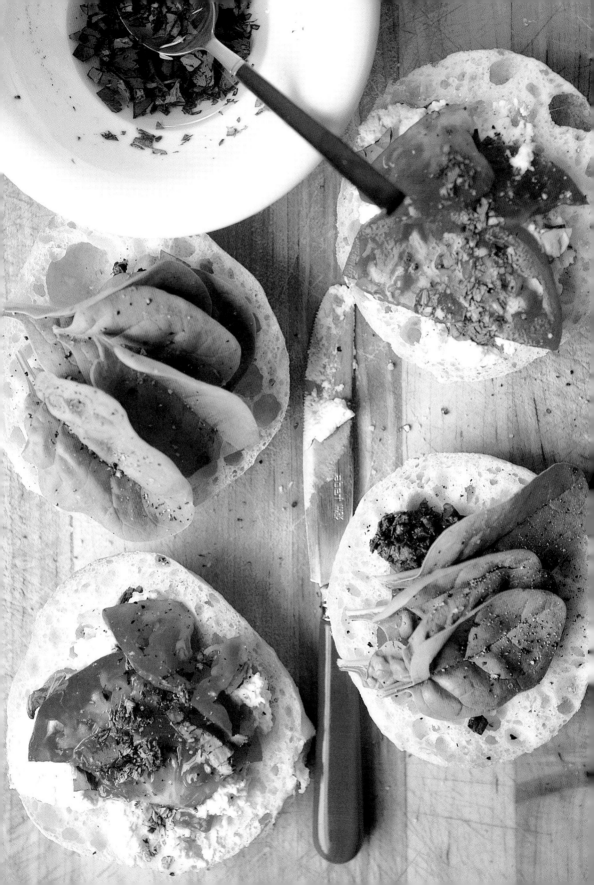

farmers' market, you can store most of them with a few drops of water in a used plastic yogurt container or in a glass container that has a snap-on lid.

Herbs are pure present tense—this moment, this day, this lunch. They are a visual and sensory signal that the meal was made right now, by hand—and in this digitalized time, that is a lot.

Use chopped parsley on anything. If it is for something hearty, such as a beef stew, you could chop it with a little garlic added. Or you can chop it with a little French salt and add that to butter or olives or even yogurt.

Basil brings youth to any tomato sauce or tomato, breadth to any soft cheese or yogurt. You can mark the very center of summer with a lunch of fresh sliced tomatoes, fresh mozzarella slices, basil leaves, salt, and olive oil—but you cannot do it without the basil.

You will be tempted to skip the chives, but they do deliver a freshness not available in any box or can. Cut the chives with scissors or a sharp knife over just about anything—even as a final touch to any soup or rice. With chives, you can make an emergency lunch of soft, spreadable cheese—even cream cheese—on crackers and be on good ground.

Mint is a luxury. Even a small spoonful of mint in rice changes everything, or a pinch in the ice water for the table. It is the warm, light wind of summer. When chopped with parsley and then added to olive oil, it makes a lovely sauce for an otherwise cold piece of leftover chicken.

Cilantro is a prerequisite for guacamole, but we now use it much more broadly. Chop cilantro into a mix with parsley and fold that into rice dishes, lentils, and soups. It has a freshness and even humor that seem always at the ready.

We will use other herbs—rosemary, thyme, sage, and dill, in particular—for many dishes cooked beforehand at home and brought in to the shop (see pages 56–105). For soups, roasts, beans, and pasta, they will be crucial. But for the moment of lunch, they are typically a bit too robust.

Sauces

There are homemade sauces aplenty that work brilliantly at lunch—from the obvious mayonnaise or tartar sauce to the subtlety of a romesco. When there is time, or on days that need the help, bringing in prepared sauces from home can be a fine relief. They are a treat but not a staple. For the daily task of lunch, we try to keep some variables as straightforward as possible.

It turns out that over a year's time, we basically use two sauces, a red and a green, never together and rarely in the same week. They are both quite hearty and wonderful, but, in truth, they only last for about three days. We keep them apart to make certain that we use each one completely.

You can use both with near abandon. Spoon some onto potato salad, mix it with avocados and green onions, or add it between the slices of any meat. The two sauces are both so buoyant and upbeat that even cold cooked fish can be dressed up. If you have some pita bread or a tortilla or a *bollo* roll that you can slightly heat, add either sauce, and then layer the bread with vegetables or meats.

Red Sauce (Salsa Roja)

MAKES ABOUT 2 CUPS.

2 green jalapeños

1 medium red onion, finely chopped

1 garlic clove, finely chopped

6 red tomatoes, peeled and roughly chopped

Juice of 1 lime

1 cup cilantro leaves, roughly chopped

Salt

Freshly ground black pepper

Most often, we buy our red salsa from a nearby Mexican grocery. They make it fresh every Monday morning. Sometimes, in the late summer when there are extra tomatoes, we will make a batch of our own.

Cut the jalapeños open, stem and seed them, and finely chop them. Add the jalapeños, onion, garlic, and tomatoes to a food processor and pulse for 20 seconds. Be careful not to over-process—you want to mix everything a bit, not pulverize the ingredients. Then add the lime juice, pulse for a moment, and add the cilantro with another quick pulse.

Taste and add salt and 2 or 3 good grinds of black pepper. Spoon the sauce into clean glass jars with tight lids and refrigerate it for up to 3 to 4 days.

Green Sauce (Salsa Verde)

MAKES ABOUT ¾ CUP.

2 or 3 bunches fresh flat-leaf parsley, washed and spun or shaken dry, stems removed

1 garlic clove

2 anchovies (optional), washed and patted dry

1 fresh, organic egg yolk (optional; skip if you cannot find a good egg)

1 teaspoon red or white wine vinegar

½ cup good olive oil

Juice of ½ lemon (optional)

Salt

This you cannot purchase and therefore must make yourself, but it is well worth the effort. It is not hard to make a good green sauce, and it will keep for three or four days. The ingredients are pretty straightforward and will make all the difference in the world to a meal. And yet few people make it. It is easy enough to see why a restaurant might steer clear: The customers would eat all of it.

Add the parsley, garlic, anchovies and egg yolk (if using), and vinegar into a food processor, pulse for a moment, and then slowly add a stream of the oil as you mix it further. You want a sauce that is clearly green and carried by, but not dominated by, the oil, so you may not need all of it. Be careful not to run the processor with abandon; it will heat and blacken the green sauce. Taste, and add salt as needed. You can also add the juice of half a lemon, to make a tarter salsa. Store in a jar with a good lid and refrigerate; bring to room temperature before serving.

SALUMI AND A GREEN SAUCE

I had not thought about a green sauce until Armandino Batali opened his salumeria in Seattle. His son, Mario, was not yet world-famous, so you could still get a table. Dino, a particularly sweet, stubborn sort, had opened Salumi on a skewed corner of Pioneer Square, a corner so obscure that even his neighbors did not know the shop was there. Once you did find it, however, you could only wish no one else would.

We would eat there three times a week, and, three times a week, he would bring out a half-finished bottle of red wine and a plate of his sliced cured meats as a welcome. Then we would start in on the meatballs and the roasted pork and the oxtail stew. But always there was green sauce about—green sauce on the sandwiches and a small glass jar of green sauce on the table. And an hour or two later, you were scraping the green sauce out of the jar with the last of the bread.

Around the holidays, when we could not get away from work but desperately needed the boost of Salumi, Dino would send up an order, with two jars of green sauce—and a note to make sure we returned the jars. Dino has since retired, and his daughter, Gina, runs Salumi brilliantly in the same skewed and now-famous location in Pioneer Square.

LAYERING

———

This is a simple but quite crucial notion. Some would call it detail or accessory or accent, but, at its best, layering is more than that: It is a touch, a finish, and it makes all the difference in the world in any cooking. For the purpose of lunch, it is quite specific: a second or third touch to what you are presenting, the signal that someone, moments before, chose and arranged and set the plate. It is personal and specific, the very first thing that people notice. The layering may be no more than a handful of parsley or chives, a grind of black pepper, a little Parmesan—all quite simply a sign of life.

You will choose the ingredients to layer by many factors—some for taste, some for color, some for the season, some for convenience, some even for humor. A lentil soup can be lightened in taste and appearance with a slice of orange and a little goat cheese on the side of the plate. A reheated pasta appears much less reluctant and more spontaneous with fresh Parmesan, parsley, and cracked pepper sitting atop it.

You must have the bits and parts on hand, they must be fresh, and you must be ready to use them. You are looking to form the proper alliances. Add color where a dish seems pale, citrus where the taste is dry, sweet where sour is unchallenged.

The layering may be horizontal, creating a more varied landscape by adding small and specific details next to what you are serving. They may be cornichons or other pickles, fig paste or cranberries, a slice of blood orange or a radish, relish or mustard, apple with mint or melon with berries, a small salad or applesauce, two slices of cheese, or a shelled walnut.

Or the layering may be vertical—building upon the structure of the dish, with elements as simple as chopped parsley or as intricate as caramelized onions and pomegranate seeds. If you have a panini press, grill day-old bread, cut it into finger-length rectangles, add a touch of olive oil, and stick the toe of each into the side of the soup just before serving. Add Parmesan last, letting it fall like snow on the soup and bread.

A Horizontal Touch

You will already have a kit of things to make this detail, the "essential foods" described in the previous pages. But you must look beyond these essentials, using the seasons as a guide. In winter, especially, look to your jars of saved fruits and vegetables, for they were each created to carry you through bare seasons. By spring, begin to add the new crops—a little rhubarb, the first peas, spring onions, or fresh herbs. And by summer, the gates open to all the fruits and vegetables.

You also have the parts from home—the not-quite-enough pasta for a meal, the few potatoes, a half spoonful of beans. Learn to scavenge your leftovers from dinners at home and restaurant meals. They are perfect actors for a smaller part.

Boiled or pan-fried potatoes: Bring the potatoes to room temperature before serving. Add a few drops of olive oil, a few drops of vinegar, black pepper, and salt. Dress them up with bits of meat or other vegetables, chopped herbs, feta mixed with olive oil, paprika, green onions, chives, yogurt with olive oil, olives, pine nuts, raisins, or other dried fruit—whatever is on hand.

Plain, cooked pasta: Bring the pasta to room temperature before serving, or micro-wave it for 30 seconds to loosen it. Add a little olive oil and a few drops of lemon juice. Do the mixing in a stainless-steel bowl—it must be tossed well and be well-loosened—then taste for salt and pepper. A chopped anchovy, some lemon zest, finely chopped broccoli, and perhaps some hot-pepper flakes are great additions. But, most import-ant, the pasta must not feel weighty or lumpy; it must be light and sprightly.

Cooked beans: You must be diligent about first letting the beans come to room temperature; like cooked potatoes and cooked pasta, they lose most of their taste in the fridge. Chopped parsley, salt, and olive oil are often all the help cooked beans need. If you also need some color, add thin slices of a cooked red pepper or slivers of salami. See pages 58–65 for more on preparing beans. A modest spoonful of beans, laid alongside a sandwich, makes both seem dressed up. The oil left behind on the plate suits the last bite of bread. Thinly chopped radishes love sitting in with the beans.

A Vertical Touch

Many of the vertical touches are also your "essential foods," but the trick is knowing how to employ them as the final finishing touch that adds a small dash of elegance to your lunch.

Flat-leaf parsley: The easiest friend, parsley makes everything taste and look fresher. When you get parsley, take its banding off and soak it for five minutes in cold water; then lift it out and spin or shake it nearly dry. Once the parsley has been washed and dried, store it in a large plastic yogurt container, stems down. It keeps for days when stored this way, fresh and crisp, and does not take on the smells of the fridge. Chop it on a clean board with a sharp knife to avoid bruising. You can also add sea salt to the parsley and chop them together to give the herb some grit and bite.

Bread crumbs, sesame seeds, peppercorns, and dried peppers: You can chop or mix any or all of these, singly, paired, or as an ensemble, and if they are fresh, they will bring immediate aid to anything, from an avocado to a soup, from a salad to a pasta.

Lemons, limes, and olive oil: These always add a breath of life to a dish, added last, with a quick toss across the surface before serving. Remember, the citrus is wet; the oil is viscous. If you are unsure which would work best, make a small pool of each and dip the food in it to taste. A taco, for example, loves lemon or lime juice and does not need olive oil. A Bolognese pasta brushes off the citrus but loves the silky olive oil.

Greens and herbs: Chives, cilantro, basil, and arugula should be chopped and usually used singly. Unlike parsley, they are not universal; they do not go well with everything. Chives love the slow-talking goat cheese or the white face of a potato; cilantro goes with avocado and lime; basil brings grace to creamy or tomato-accented pastas, soft cheeses, or warm broths. Chopping a handful of arugula and laying it across a hot soup makes the soup new again.

Cheeses: You can use grated Parmesan, of course, but also sometimes use the sharper pecorino. Or try a crumbling of *queso blanco* (a mild mozzarella) or the tangy manchego. I know a salad is ready to be served when there is a dusting of Parmesan out to its edge.

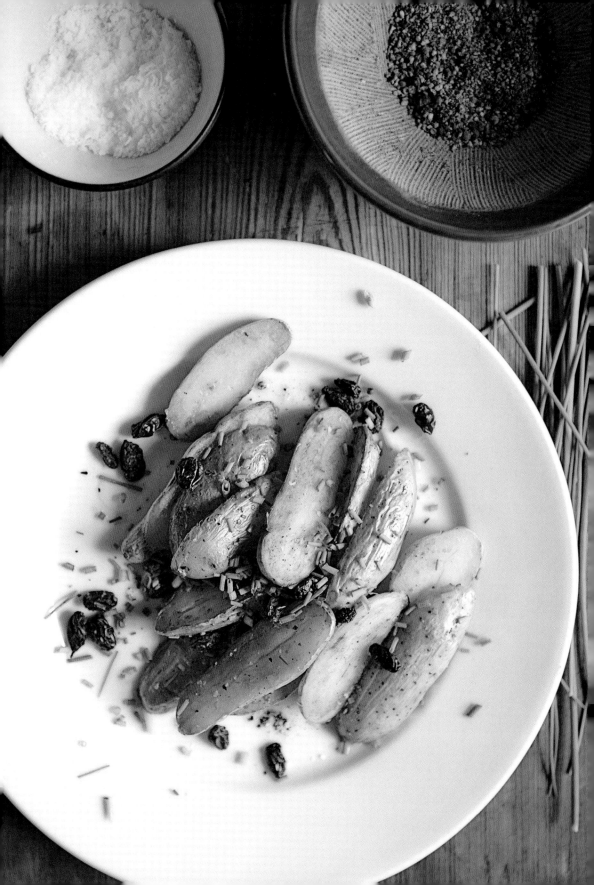

CHAPTER 2

FIRST INTENTIONS:
MEALS MADE ENTIRELY AT THE SHOP

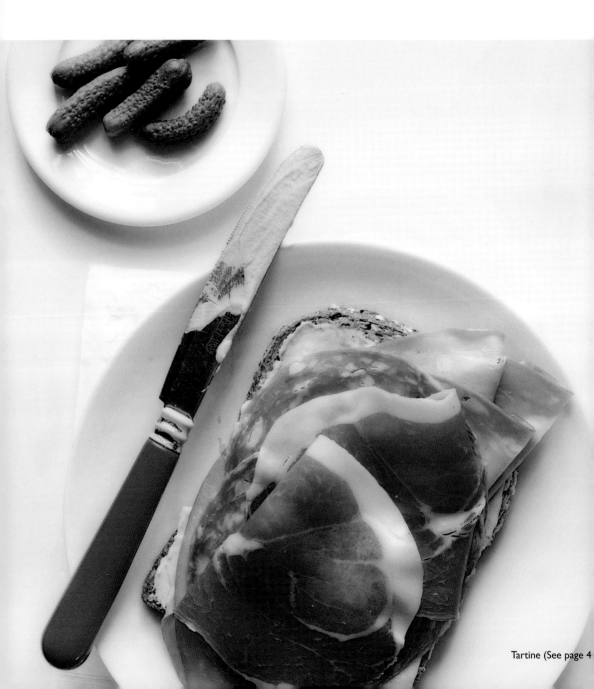

Tartine (See page 4

We have a few stalwarts, lunches that we serve at least once a month, sometimes once a week, knowing that they work and that they are a pleasure. To make these lunches, you must plan, but they are easy to make, their ingredients are easily procured, and, with a little attention, they are handsome to present. Sometimes, when we are too distracted or the ingredients are too good (spinach and a good goat cheese in the spring, for example), we will make the same sandwich for a couple of days in a row.

The following recipes are variations on the salad and the sandwich—lunch regulars. Once you have sourced your ingredients and stocked your kitchen, these lunches will take only a few minutes to prepare and can be made even in the most basic of shop kitchens. Your careful attention to detail will make each stand out and give each form and exception.

Before going on, let me say, it is *lunch*. At its simplest, it may be no more than a piece of bread, a piece of fruit, and a bit of cheese. But it is best if the bread is good, the fruit is fresh, and the cheese is true.

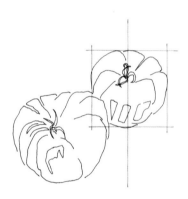

SANDWICHES OF A DIFFERENT SORT

If your lettuce is good, your avocado ready; if a lemon is on hand; if there is some roast chicken left, or any marinated onions, or good mustard; if the rolls are fresh—these are your pieces. Play them.

You are not wrapping the sandwich in plastic and letting it sit for six hours. You can be generous with heights, you can salt between the layers, your greens can stick out and even fall out; the sandwich is staying right there. Fool with it. Sweeten it with a little fig spread, loosen it with a salsa, sharpen it with a cheese or a mustard, smooth it with a butter. Making a sandwich is considerably more fun when you have a cast of extras eager to get onstage.

Tartines Wearing Many Hats

SERVES FOUR.

12 to 14 slices good country bread

½ cup (1 stick) unsalted butter, softened

2 tablespoons very good smooth French mustard

Salt

12 to 14 slices each mortadella, Genoa salami, serrano ham, and porchetta, or other cured meats

The very construction of a tartine is suited to lunch at the shop: With a two-slice sandwich, you can grab it and go, and you may never even look inside it. But to eat a tartine, you must stop for a moment and attend to it. It has no lid, it cannot be wrapped or stacked, and it can only sit upright.

It's a very simple sandwich—but, of course, it's a little tricky in its own way. With a bit of planning and care, you can make your own tartines and craft your own unique combinations. It is a fine place to start your tradition of making lunch, for it is a perfect example of the pleasure of good ingredients.

There is simply no place on a tartine to hide—everything shows, and everything matters. You must start with very good bread. This is the first important detail: a sour rye or light rye or light whole-wheat loaf will work best. The crust must give in to the bite, or the sandwich will fly apart. The butter must be soft but not melted (the French are very specific about such matters, and in this they are correct). The meat is layered gently atop the bread, not pressed or crammed shut with a top piece. What is important is the lightness of it all—that the ingredients not appear paved to the bread.

You must be attentive about a few things. The cured meat must not have stringy, inedible casing still attached, or the ham a hard gristle. The meat cannot be dried or hard to chew or still cold from the fridge. It is meant to be eaten with the bread, all together with each bite. If your guests are picking the meat off, then something has gone wrong. A tartine is eaten completely: nothing left.

Lay the bread in front of you, and butter the top face of each slice to the edges. Spread the mustard over the butter—they must merge, with neither greater than the other in strength. Sprinkle a light bit of salt on each tartine.

Layer the meat over the butter and mustard. For the mortadella, fold it gently in half; do not crease the fold. For the salami, layer the slices like tiles. Depending on its cut and size, fold or tuck each slice of ham to fit the tartine. And for the porchetta, lay two folded pieces alongside each other.

Serve each person 2 to 3 tartines, always with something on the side. It doesn't need to be complicated—a bit of fruit, a few carrots. These open-faced sandwiches can appear quite lonely on a plate, and they need a slight variation of taste to set off the flavors of the sandwich. (Cornichons or fresh pickles are perfect for the task.)

Variations: We have started with the simplest of the tartine form, but there are numerous variations on the above recipe, of course. Pâté is lovely (should you have chives, even the tiniest handful is wonderful when sprinkled over the pâté), and so is a good Brie, with perhaps some greens just below it, or avocado slices with pickled red onions.

ROLLS IN COPENHAGEN

The Danes are very specific about their lunches, and there is a remarkable, sushilike complexity to the detail of their sandwiches. In Copenhagen, there was a wonderful bakery, Kransekagehuset, up three steps on the Ny Østergade, where I often stocked up on jams and pastries before the trip back to the States. In the alley behind the bakery, they also operated a café, serving breakfast and lunch.

On one of my visits there for lunch, I was in a queue behind two elegantly dressed women who were obviously regulars, for everyone greeted them. Each sandwich at the bakery is made to order to your specifications, and as the women approached the case, I was eager to see what they would choose.

To my great surprise, their most careful consideration involved which roll to select. There was a great wicker basket of fresh rolls—at least six dozen of them—and the women considered them all, even though they were all, in theory and to me, the very same roll. Each woman chose a particular roll and then, quite quickly by comparison, decided what they would put inside the roll, before happily going off to find a table.

I had never thought to know or even bluff at knowing which roll was best. I had never given it such consideration. Now, of course, I tend to notice all the variations of a bread—how it is affected by humidity, when it is freshest, and what its best uses are.

They make a wonderful brioche at Le Pichet in Seattle. One morning, after my return from Copenhagen, there were a dozen of them on a plate, just out of the oven. I asked the young manager if one of them was the best of the lot. He laughed and said, "Of course!"

A Sandwich with Fresh Apple, *Fromager d'Affinois*, Arugula, and Almond Butter

SERVES FOUR.

8 slices of bread or 4 split rolls

4 tablespoons unsalted butter

4 tablespoons almond butter, preferably crunchy

8 ounces *Fromager d'Affinois* or Brie, sliced ½" thick

1 good handful of arugula leaves

2 in-season apples or Bosc pears, quartered, cored, and thinly sliced

Salt

2 to 3 teaspoons fresh lemon juice

This has long been a favorite at the shop and has even made the very exclusive list of "Can you make me one for my flight?" It is quite easy to put together and makes for a fine way to begin a week. It does have its specifics, a few crucial details. You must find the proper bread or roll: It can be neither too hard nor too soft, too dense nor too airy. Some bollo *rolls have worked perfectly; some dinner rolls will do, though you may end up needing to make more than one sandwich per person, due to their size. There is a baguette from a local bakery here that is perfect, except that it gets too crusty by the afternoon. Once you find the proper bread, the rest is quite simple.*

You can also use a Brie for the cheese, or a softer boursin. The Fromager d'Affinois *somehow seems to stand up best in this sandwich; it is younger than a Brie, and that youth keeps the sandwich from feeling weighty. For the best version of this sandwich, make it when the apples or pears are in season. The apple should be crisp and distinctly tasty, and that is not such an easy thing to find these days.*

It is an interesting balance: the sweet almond butter, the soft, mild cheese, with the spicy greens and the apple cutting through. Do not forget the salt — it keeps the gooey parts from having too much input.

The sandwiches might be a little tall, but if the bread is not too hard or the layers too heavy, they should hold together. This is also a dish that can be served open-faced, though it can be a challenge to stack the parts and not have them tumble over as you try to take a bite.

Butter one side of the bread slices or rolls. Spread one side of the bread slices or rolls with the almond butter. Lay one slice of cheese on the buttered side of the bread or roll. Place arugula leaves on top of the cheese (they can stick out from the edges).

Fan the apple or pear slices over the almond butter; it will help keep them in place. Sprinkle with a little bit of salt and lemon juice, and close the tartines.

The sandwiches can be made in advance and are best at room temperature, which allows the cheese to soften and its taste to mesh with the apple or pear, almond butter, butter, and greens. When you serve the sandwich, lay extra slices of the fruit on the side. Squirt some lemon juice on them so they do not brown. You can also make a simple salad with any extra arugula you have on hand, and serve it alongside.

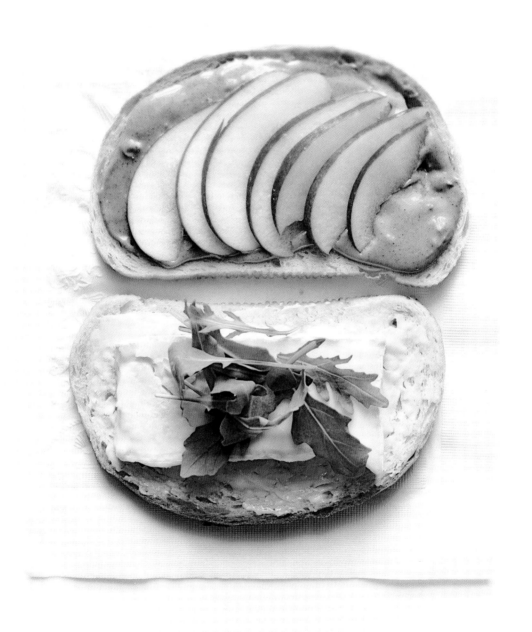

A Tuna Sandwich, Fresh with Avocado, Onion, and Horseradish

────────

SERVES FOUR.

1 small red onion, thinly sliced

1 can (8 ounces) tuna packed in olive oil

Salt

Freshly ground black pepper

1 to 2 tablespoons mayonnaise (see *Note*)

1 teaspoon horseradish, plus more as needed, if mild

½ lemon

¼ cup fresh flat-leaf parsley leaves, chopped

¼ cup fresh basil leaves, chopped

8 slices of bread

1 ripe avocado, halved, pitted, peeled, and sliced

1 tomato, cored and sliced

½ cup arugula leaves

I have eaten many a tuna sandwich, and there is a sourness in my recollection of a good half of them. This one, pictured on page 17, veers as far as possible from such a taste.

I put a few essentials into my tuna sandwich and keep a handful in mind that would love to be a part of it. It depends on what I have. But no matter what else might be involved, always buy good canned tuna packed in olive oil—the Italians are very good at this. They take their tuna, like their tomatoes, seriously. But there are many grades, and many producers, and some crooks, so you must learn who has the best fish. If you want the best, have someone bring you a can of the best grade from Peck, a lovely food shop in Milan, or any good food shop in Italy, and then you will know the taste you are hunting for. If Italy is out of reach, pick a good food store, and tell them you are in search of the best olive oil–packed tuna.

In searching for a bread for the tuna sandwich, you can range right down to Wonder Bread or well up to a dense Danish rye, which are both available in every corner store. Or try the dinner rolls now being used to make Vietnamese bánh mì *sandwiches—even hamburger buns would be fine, if they are fresh.*

Place the onions in a small bowl with enough water to cover, and set aside for 10 minutes to sweeten. Rinse the onions in cold water, and dry on a paper towel.

Drain the tuna, and place it in a large bowl. Taste the tuna—it may have been salted before canning, so do not skip this—and season with salt and pepper, as needed.

Add some mayonnaise (see *Note*)—just enough to loosen the tuna, and not so much that it becomes a *tonnato* sauce. Then add the horseradish, for bite, and a squeeze of lemon, for freshness. Taste, and season with more horseradish or lemon, as desired. Mix in the parsley and basil.

Spread some mayonnaise on one side of each slice of bread. Divide the tuna evenly among 4 slices, laying it softly on the mayonnaise. Crack some pepper and sprinkle some lemon juice on top to keep it all sprightly.

Then there are the toppings: Add a couple of avocado slices. Lightly salt the tomato slices, and place them over the avocado (but if tomatoes are not in season, this is not the time for a tasteless supermarket variety—better to skip it altogether). Pile on some arugula, to offset the moisture of the fish, and top with some of the onions. Cap each sandwich with a second slice of bread.

Cut the sandwich so that each layer can be seen; you might even let some of the greens poke out. Serve something crispy on the side— corn chips, carrots, celery, or radishes.

Note: Store-bought mayonnaise is fine, though you must ask yourself how so many eggs can sit unrefrigerated on a shelf. If you can, make your own mayonnaise at home (there are many recipes available, most of them very similar) and bring it to the office. It is not hard, and you will be controlling the freshness of the oil and the eggs.

If you prefer, you can skip the mayonnaise entirely. If you do, then in a small bowl add a little lemon juice and some salt. Let it sit for a couple of minutes, and beat in some olive oil to mix. You will need to hold aside half of the parsley and basil from the tuna and add it here to the lemon juice and olive oil. Spoon this mixture onto the bread in place of the mayonnaise.

Variation: Toppings: This version of the sandwich is a favorite of ours, but you have countless other options for toppings. Drizzle a little salsa across avocados. Try anchovies, if you can, or capers, or chopped black olives, as a simplified tapenade. What you must keep in mind are the textures and the tastes of this sandwich. When you serve it, the sea must seem fresh, the greens not waterlogged, the parts not mushed.

Tarragon: Basil and parsley are our preferred herbs, but don't limit yourself to these. Rosemary is probably too specific, but should you find fresh tarragon in the market, forgo the mayo and try mixing the tuna with a little balsamic vinegar, lemon juice, and a pinch of tarragon, and let that carry the tuna.

A Spinach Sandwich, Friends with Olive and Basil

———

SERVES FOUR.

½ pound baby spinach leaves

¼ cup olive oil

4 split *bollo* or ciabatta rolls

4 teaspoons black olive tapenade

8 ounces ricotta

1 large beefsteak tomato or 3 Roma tomatoes

10 to 12 fresh basil leaves

Salt

Freshly ground black pepper

We make this most often in the spring and fall, when the spinach seems best. But there is good year-round baby spinach now, and the sandwich is so good that we are content to make do and serve it anytime.

Tapenade is available on most grocery store shelves, but those varieties are often smooth, blended pastes. Look for freshly made tapenade instead. You must hold out for one that tastes like a wonderful olive—that taste is crucial to this sandwich. Otherwise, you can make it yourself quite easily, cutting up black olives, capers, and roasted peppers, and sometimes anchovies and garlic, and mixing it all with good olive oil. If you have some left over, tapenade makes for a wonderful end-of-day snack on a salted cracker or slice of dense rye. Ricotta, a whey cheese, comes in many varieties but must be fresh and smell fresh. We only buy what we need for sandwiches that day; it does not keep particularly well.

But the basil is the secret. If you leave it out or it has no taste, the sandwich will seem flat.

You can grill this on a panini press if you have one, though it takes some care to not make a mess. It is wonderful as is, a fine tribute to ingredients working together. It can be made an hour early if you cover the sandwiches with wax paper and do not refrigerate.

Wash the spinach well, even if it is loose, and *very* well if it is not. Critters and sand love spinach. Using the biggest bowl you have, soak the spinach in cool water, then carefully lift it out, change the water, and repeat until the water is clear. Then spin the spinach or lay it on dishtowels to dry; it must be dry for this dish.

Spread the oil on both split surfaces of each roll. Spread the tapenade on one side of each roll, and the ricotta on the other side.

Cut the tomato into 4 horizontal slices, and lay one slice on the ricotta side of each roll. Tear the basil leaves and lay them over the tomatoes, distributing them evenly among the sandwiches. Lay 3 tiers of the spinach leaves (about 10 to 12 leaves of the baby spinach total, maybe only 4 to 5 if the leaves are bigger), curled downward, over the tomato on each roll. It should almost totter with spinach, loosely laid. Season both sides with salt and pepper and close the rolls. (Salt is crucial to this sandwich, as it keeps all the parts in play, but be careful to avoid oversalting—the tapenade can already be salty.)

Serve the sandwiches with something to crunch, such as a sliced radish or a carrot or some plain chips.

———

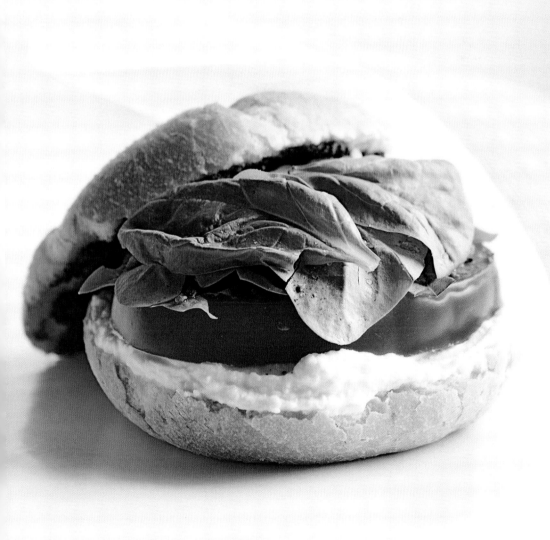

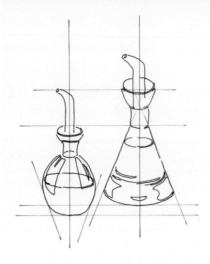

A SALAD TO STAND ALONE

It is not easy to serve a salad for lunch at the shop. Yes, if it is summer and you have truly fresh tomatoes, basil, peas, young onions, and lovely greens, then you can trust the tastes and color of the season to carry the meal. But for much of the year, the greens are not spry, and the tomatoes are a bit haggard, and that makes a salad a braver task.

For such times, you must lean on your ingredients. Soaking the greens in cold water for five minutes can bring them nearly back to life (limp basil may take a few more minutes than that). Spin the greens dry and lay them in a bowl with a dishtowel over it. And then consider how to make a silk purse from these sows' ears.

In truth, you should be able to make a salad that easily outdoes at least the premade salads in clear plastic boxes that are stacked in the grocery cooler. Regardless of season or urban supply, you have apples that can be jumbled with blue cheese, sliced meats that can be brightened up with a green sauce or a romesco, and tuna that can be tossed with cherry tomatoes. If you take the few moments needed to mix the parts in sequence—not just simply jumble them all together—you can give a salad depth and complexity.

Your strength is preparation and materials: good oil and vinegar, true peppercorns, French salt, hopefully an herb or two, garlic that has not gone soft, Parmesan made in Italy, fresh feta. The quality of your ingredients is a true advantage and the hand you need to play.

Whether the salad is plain or weighty with components, if it is the main course, serve it on a larger plate. That will leave room for accessories, and the accessories, of course, will make all the difference. Add olives to what is left of the dressing and lay them around the salad—or cherry tomatoes and crumbled feta, in the same bowl, spooned in at the side. A spoonful of fig jam or a chutney, perhaps on a couple of crackers, or some goat cheese with olive oil and pepper. Use what you like; fool with what you have. The alley around the salad is yours for fun, for color, a kind of bazaar of tastes and textures, and you can lay a small marketplace of bites and pieces out to escort the now proud salad.

A Very Good Basic Vinaigrette

MAKES ABOUT ⅓ CUP.
TO DRESS A SALAD FOR FOUR.

And of course, for any salad, begin with a very good dressing.

In your serving bowl, dissolve the salt in the vinegar for a couple of minutes. Then, with a fork, whisk in the oil and 1 teaspoon of water until emulsified. The water helps to pull the dressing together. Then taste—you may need more oil, if the vinegar is still sharp, or more salt, if the salt is mild.

Once the base of the dressing is mixed, you can tip in some garlic or herbs. You can thin and acidify it with a few drops of lemon or lime juice, or thicken and hearten it with a little cream, mustard, or yogurt. Whisk the additions in with a fork to combine.

Salt, to taste

1 tablespoon red or white wine vinegar

5 to 6 tablespoons olive oil

Optional:

1 clove garlic, crushed

1 tablespoon chopped fresh herbs

Fresh lemon or lime juice

1 teaspoon heavy cream

1 teaspoon mustard

1 teaspoon Greek yogurt

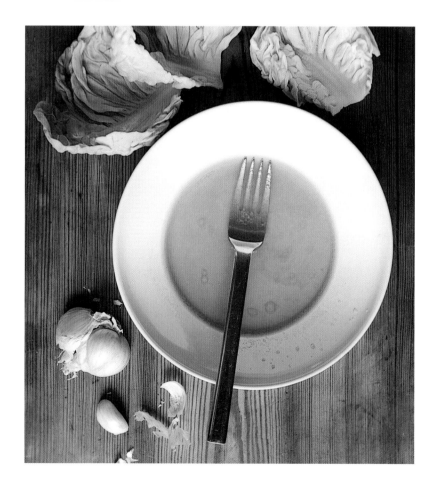

Caesar Salad: A Noble Reinforcement

SERVES FOUR.

I head romaine lettuce

I anchovy fillet

I clove garlic, minced

½ teaspoon Worcestershire sauce

I teaspoon salt

Juice of I lemon, squeezed halves reserved

I egg yolk

3 tablespoons olive oil

Freshly ground black pepper

½ cup freshly grated Parmesan cheese

I cup freshly made croutons

If your only greens are the stiff-collared romaine, then you may be best served by presenting the meal of a Caesar salad—one that will coat and cover and fill, and that can be constructed out of a larder of ingredients, some of which the shop kitchen will already have on hand.

Caesar is a stuffy, much-abused dressing, but if you make your own, if you keep a light touch, if you do not use it like a coat of plaster, then it can bail out a bowl of greens. It was quite a good idea once, until it was overloaded and became more of a cover than a subtlety.

You must taste the lemon and pepper in the dressing, and almost taste the garlic and Worcestershire. And this is not the time to use pre-grated Parmesan—it is grated too thickly and is often too gummy. Use a fine grater and good Parmesan, even a slightly dry piece; you want almost a powder of the cheese.

If you have a burner or oven or stove top, then you can prepare the croutons at work. If you do not, settle for a day-old variety that you can bring in from home. Tear some bread (even a hamburger/hotdog roll will do!) into small pieces, put them in a bowl, drizzle a little olive oil over the top, add salt and pepper, and pour them out onto a sauté pan or cookie sheet. Put the sheet into an oven preheated to 400 °F or the pan on a burner set to medium heat, and brown them. Keep a close watch so that they do not burn, stirring or shaking often. Know that if you leave warm, browned croutons out on the counter, some-one will eat them before they get to any salad.

Make sure the lettuce is clean and dry. In your serving bowl, mash the anchovy and garlic together with a fork to just combine. Add the Worcestershire, salt, and lemon juice, stirring as you go.

In a small bowl, stir the yolk to break it up a bit, and pour it into the anchovy mixture, stirring with the fork to combine. When it is all blended, stir the oil into the dressing, and keep stirring until it is emulsified. You must taste the dressing—it is crucial that it not go past the point of tartness. When the taste is to your liking, then add the lettuce, and toss to coat. Season with pepper, top with the cheese, and, at the very last moment, add a bit more lemon by squeezing the spent halves. It works if it is not cloying.

Place the salad on individual plates, and then toss the croutons into the dressing remaining in the empty salad bowl before dividing them among the plates. For a salad so dense with flavors, should you want something at the side of the plate, add apple or pear slices or navel orange pieces—anything that will not add to the congestion of tastes.

A Salad with Plenty of Parts

SERVES FOUR.

6 ounces goat cheese

1 head Bibb lettuce or red- or green-leaf lettuce

2 lemons

Salt

¼ cup olive oil, plus more as needed

1 small dried red chili pepper

1 bunch fresh cilantro or flat-leaf parsley, finely chopped

1 ripe avocado, halved, pitted, peeled, and sliced

Freshly ground black pepper

6 ounces marinated vegetables (broccoli, cauliflower) or rice or orzo salad

4 ounces pickled sliced red onions (see *Note*)

Plain crackers or rye bread

This is a salad for days of less bounty. It will work year-round but is a particular help when greens are sparse and the days are gray. It is a way of making do with a very short shopping list and an even shorter choice of fresh vegetables. Most grocery stores will have some version of a rice or orzo salad or marinated vegetables in their refrigerated case; this is simply a recipe to use them and dress them up a bit.

It is the disparate parts that make this salad work and that bring it to life—the quickness of the lemon, the thin line of the cilantro, the bite of the chili, the slightly sour smoothness of the goat cheese, and then the marinated vegetables against the avocado. The avocado should be ripe enough that you can slice it with a butter knife.

It is a salad of layering and parts. As such, it first takes a little shopping, then a few minutes of prepping. Get everything laid out and organized—when it is ready to go, you must move quickly. All the parts must appear as if they have only just arrived, a little out of breath. It is the spontaneity of this salad that makes it such a pleasure.

Open the goat cheese to let it soften.

Make sure the lettuce is clean and dry. Tear the largest leaves in half, but keep the smaller ones whole.

Juice one of the lemons into a small bowl and add a good pinch of salt. Let it sit for a couple of minutes until the salt starts to dissolve (you start with the acid of the lemon because salt does not dissolve in oil, a fat). Then, stirring with a fork, add the oil and a couple of drops of cold water.

Pour a bit of oil into a teacup (about 2 tablespoons), and, with your fingers, crush a small bit of the dried chili into the oil to taste, and save the rest for another meal. (Make sure to wash your hands thoroughly after handling the chili, and avoid touching your eyes.) Add 1 tablespoon of the cilantro to the oil.

Lay the avocado in a medium bowl, and squeeze the juice from half of the remaining lemon over them. Mash the avocado and lemon juice with a fork to just combine. Keep it lumpy—you are not trying to make a smooth paste. Add half of the remaining cilantro, and salt and black pepper to taste, and stir slightly.

Place the greens in a large stainless-steel bowl, sprinkle a tiny bit of salt over them, add the dressing, and toss well to coat. Spread the greens among four plates, taking care that if they are cupped, you have them facing upward. Evenly divide the avocado mixture among the plates, placing it over one-third of the lettuce. Add the marinated vegetables or rice or orzo salad quickly to the empty dressing bowl to moisten them with the dressing that remains, and then divide among the plates, placing them next to the avocado over one-third of the lettuce. Finish each plate by placing a small scoop of the goat cheese over the final third of the greens.

Sprinkle more cilantro over the avocado mixture on each plate, lay 2 or 3 rings of the pickled onions over the vegetables or rice, and drizzle a tiny bit of the oil infused with hot pepper over the goat cheese. Squeeze a few drops of lemon juice from the remaining lemon half over each plate just before serving.

Serve the salad with unflavored fresh crackers or slices of dense rye bread—whichever you choose, make sure they are spread with good butter. (See opposite for the salad in the process of being made, and page 8 for the finished product.)

Note: To pickle onions yourself: Thinly slice a small red onion, and then put it in a small bowl with a pinch of salt, enough white wine vinegar to moisten it all, a teaspoon of sugar, and some cracked black pepper. Let this sit, covered with a plate, for 20 minutes (or longer, if you have the time and think of it earlier in the day, though even a few minutes is time enough to pickle the onions a bit).

———————————

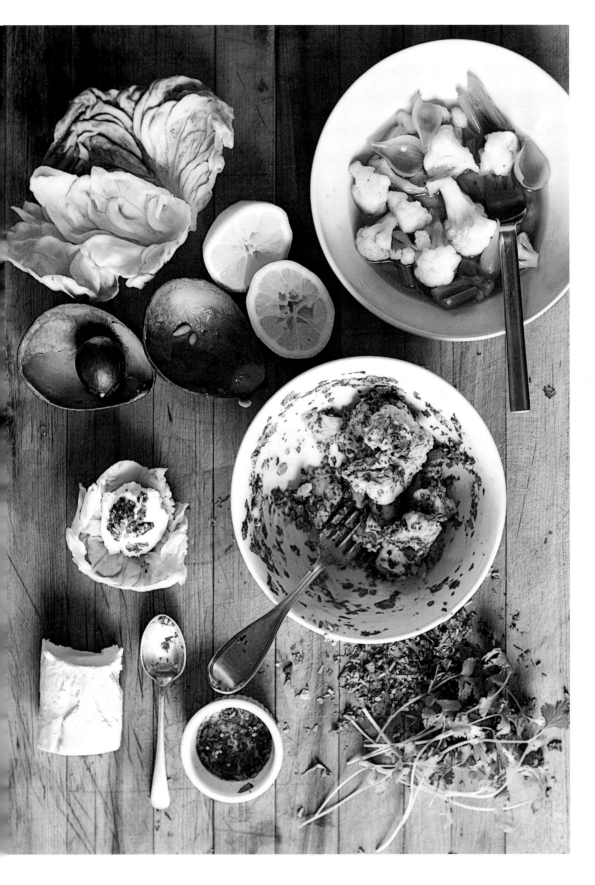

CHAPTER 3

THE FORMIDABLE ALLY OF HOME:
A BIT FROM HERE, A BIT FROM THERE

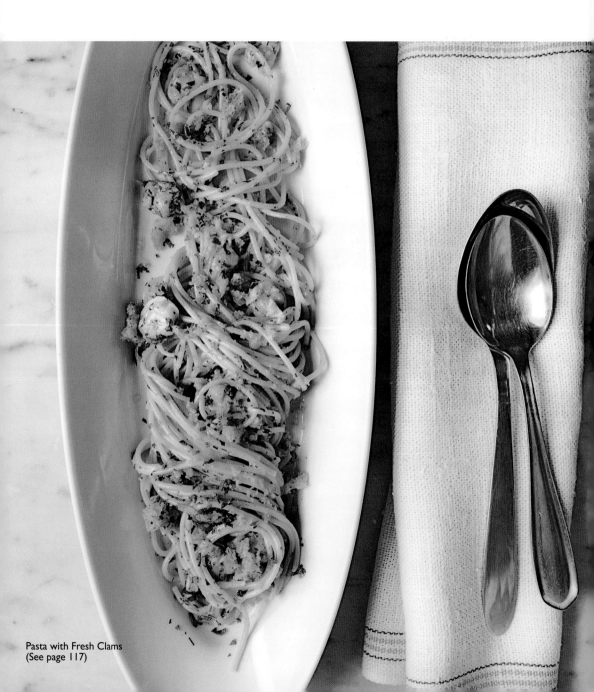

Pasta with Fresh Clams
(See page 117)

We are all busy. It is too much to expect people to make an entire lunch at home every day and cart it into work. It is far easier to look for parts and pieces, to make a bit more pasta carbonara for dinner and save it, knowing how well it will combine with a simple chicken soup the next day. You will not be bringing lunch from home—you will be bringing the parts for lunch from home.

With a bit of planning and attention, you can use the time and materials of making dinner to your advantage. The dishes in this chapter need prepping at home, but their components are quite straightforward—they are meant to be. They can be made while you are otherwise cooking, or even while you are doing dishes.

Lunch will utilize the bits of parsley, the quarter cup of gravy, the chicken that is not enough for a sandwich. Lunch will employ the small handful of pasta, the spoonful of risotto, the lone hamburger. The stray parts will find their way into soups, lentils, rice, beans, or plain linguine.

The recipe instructions are written under the assumption that you will use your home kitchen to handle the initial stages of each recipe—those tasks that need an oven or a stove top or extra time—and then finish the recipe at work. For example, the first stages of a good soup will often require an hour or two of simmering the broth, and this can easily be done at home, even while you are doing other tasks. But finishing the preparation and serving the soup, adding the basil and the fresh Parmesan cheese and bits of fresh pasta—these steps can be done at work. It will give the soup a true and obvious freshness.

However, if you wish, complete the preparation of a dish entirely at home, and serve it right away. You still can bring in whatever is left and serve it for lunch the next day. At work, you have parsley, olive oil, lemon, freshly ground pepper, and assorted condiments to help refresh the dish and give it an air of immediacy.

Beans and lentils, pasta and rice are what we call the mortar of lunch, and they will be discussed in detail throughout this chapter. Once you learn their manner and their range, you will always want to have them on hand. They are wonderful alone or combined with one another. They love playing with other flavors. They can sit beside a meal or below a meal, or they can *be* the meal. Here we include a few of our favorite basic methods of preparation as well as recipes that make use of these four essentials in different ways, hinting at the unlimited possibilities they offer. In addition, this chapter focuses on meats, from fish to beef, offering different ways of prepping at home in order to make use of them the next day. All these primary ingredients must come from a proper kitchen, for they take a little time and some preparation and require pots and pans and a stove top.

The truth is, lunch is best when it is related to the dinners that came before. In the short time and limited space of making lunch at the shop, you must be ingenious and vigilant about your presentations. With a bit of planning, imagination, and humor, there will be no talk about leftovers. But everyone will talk about lunch.

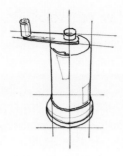

BEANS

You must learn to make beans a habit. They are easy and ample and wonderful if you keep them in mind, but grumpy and slow and inflexible if you do not. They need to be soaked for at least ten hours, overnight if you can, in cold water, and the water must be refreshed as the beans expand so that they are always covered. Cover the pot or bowl in which the beans are soaking so that nothing can fall in with them. If you forget to soak the beans in advance, there are tricks to make up for lost time. But I suggest you make something else and remember to soak the beans another day.

I will often cook beans a day or two in advance, while I am making dinner or just after—they do not take much attention, but they do take a little time. Once you have them cooked, they will last nearly a week in the refrigerator. You may not have a specific idea for them, but a day later, they may be just the thing to carry or bolster a meal.

The dried white, red, green, and brown kinds sit on the shelves of every grocery story from Alaska to the Florida Panhandle. But their packaging is hardly ever dated and rarely includes information about where the beans were grown. There is little left in the modern world of dried bean traditions. But know that all beans are not the same—and that beans dried, bought, and cooked within a year are better than beans from King Tut's tomb. There are many vendors that will mail you dried beans and lentils. We use Purcell Mountain Farms in Idaho (www.purcellmountainfarms.com). When I lay out a cup of their cannellini beans, virtually none of them are broken or browned. Purcell Mountain grows and sells them within the harvest year. Similarly, their lentils are harvested and sold within a calendar year.

On one hand, I would urge you to simply push forward and begin to learn about and cook beans. But on the other, I urge you to show them great respect and honor. They are true royalty. They have survived neglect, elitism, modernism, and casual ignorance. Their production is sustainable, their tastes are elegant, and their value, in terms of health, is unassailable.

Each recipe in this section has a slightly different course, achieving a distinct effect: a red bean cooked with vegetables, a white bean cooked with garlic, a fresh bean barely cooked at all. Cooking with them is a bit like learning to play the piano: The start is quite manual, but complexity and richness are up ahead.

One Way to Cook Beans

SERVES FOUR.

At home:

2 cups dried beans, soaked overnight

Salt

Optional:

1 bay leaf

1 clove garlic

1 sprig thyme

1 celery stalk

½ onion

Beans took a turn toward obscurity in the early 1950s. They stood around looking unmodern in a world that wanted very much to move ahead and be modern. But now they are back, and their subtleties are being celebrated in very celebrated restaurants. Here is a straightforward way to cook dried beans. After you cook them—then it gets interesting.

At home: Rinse the beans, picking through them and tossing any broken pieces away. Put them in a saucepan with 6 cups of cold water, plus more as needed to cover the beans. Do not add salt until after they are cooked, but throw in a bay leaf, garlic, thyme, celery, or onion—toss any or all in, as they are; there's no need to chop them.

Bring the water to a slow boil over medium to medium-high heat. Stir at the start, until the boiling liquid keeps the beans moving. Then turn the heat down to low, just enough to keep the slowest boil. Leave the pot uncovered. If any foam collects on the surface, skim it away. Add more water as needed to keep the beans covered as they cook.

The beans should be done in 45 to 60 minutes, but the many variations in bean size and age will affect cooking time, and some can take up to 2 hours to cook. Taste them every 10 minutes or so after 45 minutes. The beans should be tender but not mushy. If you must err on any side of doneness, however, err toward soft rather than tough. You can always make a pureed soup.

Once the beans are tender, then you can add some salt. Discard the herbs, garlic, celery, and onions—their job is done (in particular, discard the bay leaf, or its flavor will overtake the taste of the beans). Keep your fingers out of the beans. The cooked beans are extraordinarily sensitive to the bacteria on your hands.

Refrigerate the beans, with their cooking liquid, in an airtight container if they are not being used right away; they will keep for up to a week. Or drain and use the beans to make one of many soups.

Cranberry Bean Soup with Vegetables and Perhaps Pasta

SERVES FOUR.

A perfectly straightforward soup made notable by how wonderful it tastes. The vegetables must cook until they sweeten, the tomato must cook until it has broken down and amalgamated, and then the cranberry beans (also called borlotti) must cook and take on extra flavor. Much of the subtlety is instilled in those first twenty minutes of preparation, then replayed each time you serve the soup.

This soup is meant to gather assorted and even homeless parts. It is a wonderful base. You could stir in small bits of meat or chicken, you could sauté some chanterelles with finely chopped onion and lay them over the soup, or you might brown some slices of bread in olive oil and poke them into the side of the bowl.

At home: In a soup pot over medium heat, heat the oil. Add the onions and cook for 5 minutes, until softened; do not let the mixture brown. Add the carrots and celery and stir well. Season with salt and pepper, stir again, and add the tomatoes (with juice). Stir to combine. Reduce the heat to low, and cook, uncovered, for 10 minutes.

Add the beans to the vegetable-tomato mixture and cook for 2 to 3 minutes. Cover the pot and cook over low heat to bring the tastes together. The mixture should be bubbling, but not madly. Stir occasionally; you do not want the beans to stick to the pot or burn. After 6 minutes, uncover the soup and stir. Scoop out a ladleful of beans and process them through a ricer into a bowl. Add ½ cup of the stock, and mix to combine. The mashed beans and stock will act as a thickener, which will bind and smooth the soup. Return the mashed-bean mixture to the pot, and continue to cook for 10 minutes, stirring. Add the remaining stock as needed, between 1 to 2 cups, adding more or less depending on whether you want a thinner or thicker soup.

Taste and season with salt and pepper. You could stop at this point and serve the soup immediately, with chopped parsley on top. Or let it cool a bit and store it in an airtight container for the next day.

At the shop: Warm the soup and taste it for seasoning, adding more salt and pepper if you see fit. Sprinkle with parsley just before serving.

Variation: Add a cup or so more stock (or even hot water!), and, keeping the soup at a slow boil, add a handful of rice or any sort of pasta, from tiny macaroni to broken ribbons. Cook until the rice or pasta is done. With rice, that should be about 15 minutes; with dried pasta, allow 8 to 10 minutes, depending on size and type.

At home:

¼ cup olive oil

1 small yellow onion, finely chopped

1 to 2 carrots, finely chopped

1 celery stalk, finely chopped

Salt

Freshly ground black pepper

½ cup diced fresh or canned peeled tomatoes

1 cup dried cranberry beans (borlotti), cooked and drained (see page 59)

3 cups warm chicken or vegetable stock

At the shop:

Salt

Freshly ground black pepper

½ cup fresh flat-leaf parsley leaves, chopped

A Lovely White Bean Soup
with Garlic and Sausage

SERVES FOUR.

Once I have cannellini beans cooked and saved in the refrigerator, all sorts of meals come to mind. Our butcher was laying out fresh sausages, and I could imagine them, cooked and charred, sticking partway out of a bowl of white beans, parsley, and black pepper.

This is a soup that needs good parsley, and plenty of it.

At home: Heat a small sauté pan over medium heat for a moment. Add 1 tablespoon of the oil, and heat for 1 minute. Add the sausage to the pan. The heat must be lively enough that they sizzle but not so intense that they burn—adjust it accordingly. Cook the sausages for 6 to 8 minutes, turning them several times while they brown and cook through (see *Note*). Remove them from the pan with a slotted spoon, and set them aside on paper towels to drain.

In a soup pot, heat the remaining ¼ cup of the oil and the garlic over medium heat. The temperature must be high enough to lightly cook the garlic but not so high that the garlic browns—reduce the heat to medium-low, if necessary. Cook, stirring occasionally and keeping careful watch, until it is aromatic, 2 to 3 minutes. (If you brown the garlic, start over; the heat was too high, and the burnt taste will ruin the delicate soup.)

Add the beans, stirring them into the oil and garlic. Season with some salt and pepper, and cover the pan. You want the aromas to infuse the beans. Cook the beans, covered, for 3 minutes, and then stir in ½ cup of the stock.

Using a slotted spoon, remove about one-third of the beans and process them through a ricer back into the pan. This will thicken the soup. Gradually add the remaining ¾ cup stock to the mix, stirring and keeping the mixture at a simmer. The warm stock will loosen the soup, so add more or less to reach the consistency you desire. You will find the balance of the whole beans and the mashed beans and the liquid—that is your soup. Taste and season with salt and pepper, add the sausage and the parsley, and stir to combine.

The soup will keep in an airtight container in the refrigerator for 3 to 5 days.

At the shop: When you reheat the soup at work, add 2 tablespoons of water to loosen its surface, then stir the soup to combine

At home:

¼ cup plus 1 tablespoon olive oil

2 mild Italian sausages sliced into 1" rounds

2 cloves garlic, finely chopped

2 cups dried cannellini beans, cooked and drained (see page 59)

Salt

Freshly ground black pepper

1 cup warm chicken stock

½ cup fresh flat-leaf parsley leaves, chopped

At the shop:

2 tablespoons olive oil

everything evenly. Drizzle the top with a thin line of the oil just before serving.

Serve the soup with slices of soft white bread to sop it up, or serve it at room temperature as a side dish to a salad.

Note: Alternatively, preheat the oven to 375°F. Coat the sausages lightly in oil, place them on a rimmed baking sheet or roasting pan, and bake for 25 minutes. Do not prick the sausages—you want them to cook from within. Let them cool before slicing them into rounds.

———————————

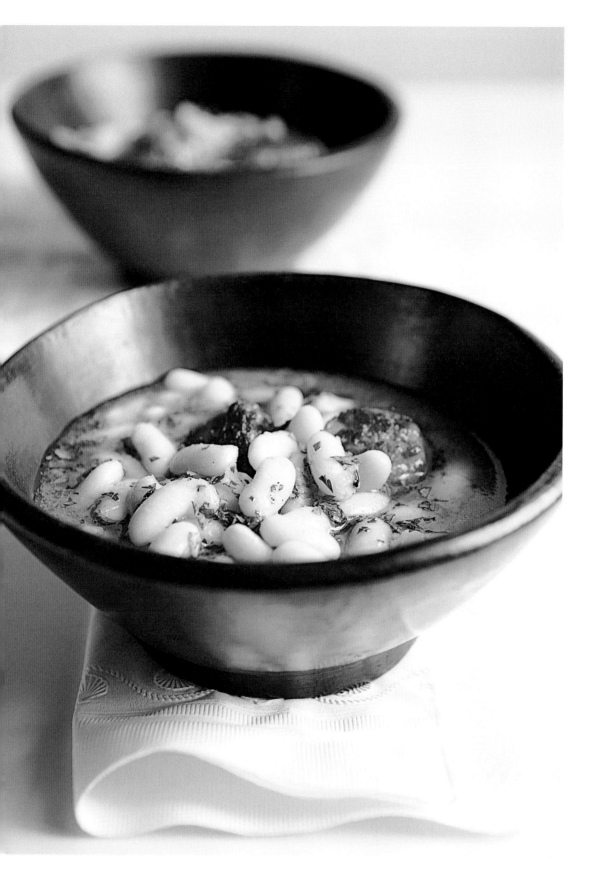

A Summer Soup with Fresh Beans, in Season

SERVES FOUR.

At home:

1 cup shelled fresh cannellini, kidney, or cranberry beans (from about 2 to 3 pounds unshelled beans)

1 bay leaf

3 cloves garlic

Salt

¼ cup olive oil

Freshly ground black pepper

1 cup warm chicken stock

At the shop:

½ cup fresh flat-leaf parsley leaves, chopped

Freshly ground black pepper

In late summer, you can often buy fresh beans in their pods or shelled, usually from a farmers' market. The pods do not look especially fresh, and even the beans themselves can look a little wan but make a point to buy them. They take all of the summer to ripen and then are dried or gone in a fortnight. Cannellini, kidney, and cranberry beans are particularly wonderful when they are fresh. They have an immediacy, a quicker, earthy smell, a softer texture.

At home: Rinse the fresh beans well—they are handled considerably while being shucked. (They do not, of course, need any soaking.) Put the beans in a saucepan with enough fresh water to cover them by 3 or 4 inches. Add the bay leaf and 1 clove of the garlic. Bring to a boil over medium heat, stirring occasionally so the beans do not stick to the pan, and then let the mixture simmer until the beans are just soft. This may take as little as 15 minutes or up to 30 minutes, depending on the size and age of the beans, so taste a bean or two after 15 minutes and every few minutes after that, until they are soft.

Turn off the heat, and remove and discard the bay leaf and garlic clove. Add some salt, to taste. Once cooled, the beans can be refrigerated in their liquid for 3 to 4 days.

In a sauté pan, heat the oil over low heat. Finely chop the remaining 2 garlic cloves and add them to the pan. Cook for 1 minute, then add the drained beans and stir to combine. Season with salt and pepper, and cover the pan. Cook for 4 to 5 minutes, letting the beans mingle intimately with the garlic. The low heat should be enough to keep them slightly bubbling, but stir if you need to—you do not want them to stick.

Uncover the pan, stir the beans, and add ½ cup of the stock to loosen the mixture. If you wish, scoop out half of the beans and process them through a ricer back into the pan to smooth and thicken the mixture. Add the remaining stock to the pan until you have reached the desired consistency, using more or less depending on how thin or thick you want your soup to be. Then taste the soup, and season, as needed, with salt and pepper.

Serve immediately, or let the soup cool, store it in an airtight container, and refrigerate it for the next day. The soup will keep for to 3 to 5 days.

At the shop: Reheat the soup, adding a little water to loosen it. Just before serving, finish the soup with chopped parsley and black pepper. Serve the soup with a piece of bread, brushed with a little oil and grilled.

Variation: If you are looking for a noteworthy addition to this recipe, buy a half rack of baby back pork ribs, cut them until they are nearly separate, and rub them with oil and salt and pepper. Preheat the oven to 400°F and put the ribs in a shallow roasting pan. Roast the ribs for 45 to 60 minutes, turning them once after 15 minutes. They should be well-browned; if not, let them cook another 15 to 20 minutes. Pull them out of the oven and cut them into single ribs. Either serve immediately or let them cool and then refrigerate them in an airtight container. At the shop, bring the ribs to room temperature, then add them to the hot bean soup just before serving—one or two ribs in each bowl, sticking up.

———

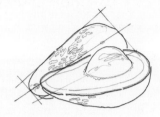

LENTILS

The difficulty of lentils is simply remembering them, for they have scant tradition in modern times. Lentils are a noble assistant to many foods and a trusty backpack to many vegetables. I make them at least once a week, every week, and use them in different proportions over many preparations: as a soup, an hors d'oeuvre, a side dish, or an underlayer to fish or pork. They "play well with others," as the saying goes. In truth, the lentil suffers when served alone; it much prefers to be part of a soup, joined with a sauce, merged with rice, topped with avocado, or tucked into vegetables.

Most often, I use the small green Puy lentils (also called French lentils) or Castelluccio lentils, an Italian variety, but there are many kinds, each a bit different, and each is very important and adored somewhere on this Earth.

You should soak them for twenty minutes before cooking, but at the very least rinse them—they get handled many times, and that alone should inform you of the necessity.

Here are three ways to cook lentils, each method a little different and suited for different occasions and ways of serving, along with a few specific recipes that will allow you to test out these methods to delicious effect.

One Way to Cook Lentils

SERVES FOUR.

At home:

1 cup lentils, soaked

1 bay leaf or sprig fresh thyme

1 teaspoon salt

This is the simplest way of cooking lentils. It can be started before you are even certain how you will use them. If I'm using a lentil with which I'm unfamiliar, I always start with this method—you will get a clear sense of their texture and smell. This way is also best if you are in a rush, as it requires less time than the methods on pages 70 and 73.

At home: Place the lentils in a small soup pot and add the bay leaf or thyme sprig and enough cold water to cover the lentils by 1 inch. Do not salt the water. Bring the water to a boil over medium-high heat, stirring so the lentils stay loose. Reduce the heat to low to maintain a gentle boil, and cook, uncovered, for 25 to 35 minutes, until the lentils are soft but before they get too mushy.

Remove and discard the bay leaf or thyme sprig. Drain the lentils in a colander, and rinse them under cool water. Put them in a bowl, add the salt, and let cool. Store them in an airtight container in the refrigerator, to be used later to create a variety of dishes, such as Lentils Folded into Yogurt, Spinach, and Basil (see page 68). They will keep for 5 to 7 days.

Variation: For a quick side dish, put the still-warm lentils into a small bowl. Mix 1 clove of minced garlic and a handful of chopped parsley with the lentils until well-combined. Taste for salt, add a good drizzle of oil and some Parmesan, and serve. If there is any left over, it will be just as good the next day, served at room temperature.

Lentils Folded into Yogurt, Spinach, and Basil

―――――――

SERVES FOUR.

Make this with a light touch so you can taste the different ingredients involved. And serve it in smaller portions than you might imagine—let people come back for seconds. It is a nod to pesto and a salute to yogurt.

You can buy baby spinach year-round. But if it is spring, buy true baby spinach, the smaller leaves of the early variety; they will have a subtler taste and texture. Wash and dry either type well; the leaves will not chop or tear cleanly if still damp.

At home:

½ cup pine nuts or chopped walnuts

2 cups baby spinach

1 cup fresh basil leaves

1 cup cooked lentils (see page 67)

2 tablespoons fresh flat-leaf parsley leaves, chopped

1 garlic clove, finely chopped

1 lemon

1 cup Greek yogurt

¼ cup olive oil

Salt

Freshly ground black pepper

At the shop:

½ lemon

½ cup Parmesan cheese, sliced

Freshly ground black pepper

Salt

At home: Heat a small sauté pan over medium heat. Add the pine nuts or walnuts and cook until lightly toasted, 5 to 7 minutes. Lay them out on a wooden cutting board to cool, then chop them roughly to the size of the lentils.

If your knife is sharp enough to slice the spinach and basil leaves without bruising them, gently cut them into bite-size pieces. Otherwise, tear them by hand.

Place the lentils in a bowl and mix in the spinach, basil, parsley, and garlic. Squeeze the lemon into the lentils, mix, and then fold in the yogurt. Mix again, then slowly pour in the oil, stirring, as you do, to combine. At this point, taste the mixture, and season with salt and 2 good grindings of pepper. Finally, fold the roasted nuts into the dish, and finish with a drizzle of oil. The dish is now ready to serve.

The lentils and greens will keep in an airtight jar or container in the refrigerator for at least 3 days.

At the shop: For lunch, bring the lentils and greens close to room temperature before serving. They can go on a slice of buttered (and perhaps grilled) bread, or on a lettuce leaf as a salad. Top the lentils with a squeeze of lemon juice, some Parmesan, and a final grind of fresh pepper.

Sometimes, if there are any lentils left after lunch, we serve them as a late-day snack, with a little extra salt at the end.

―――――――

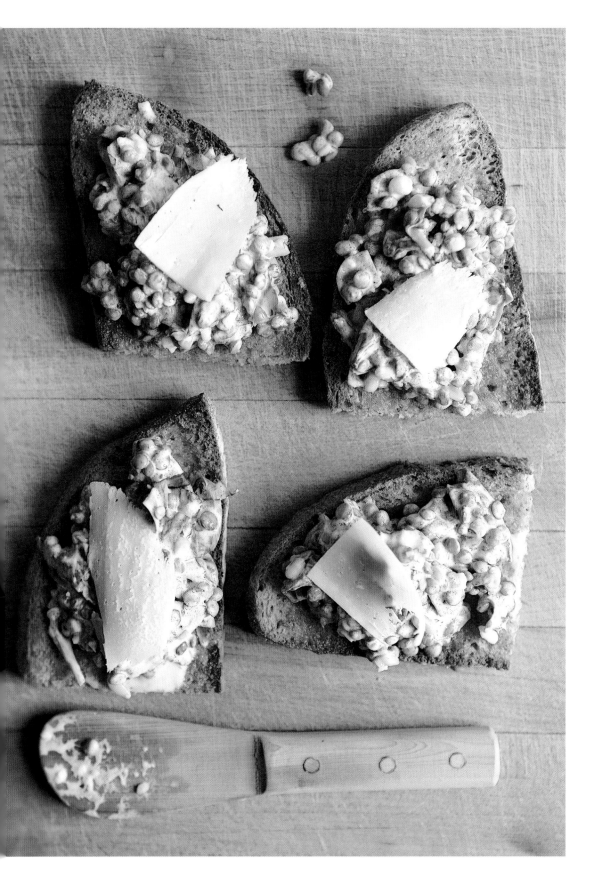

A Second Way to Cook Lentils

SERVES FOUR.

This method is more intricate than the first, akin to making risotto but without the constant stirring. It takes five to ten minutes more, but it has a subtler result.

At home:

3 tablespoons olive oil

1 yellow onion, finely chopped

1 piece (3 ounces) pancetta or guanciale (optional)

1 carrot, finely chopped

1 celery stalk, finely chopped

1 cup lentils, soaked and drained

1 sprig fresh rosemary

1 bay leaf

6 to 8 cups warm chicken or vegetable stock

4 tablespoons (¼ cup) cold butter

2 tablespoons fresh flat-leaf parsley leaves, chopped

Salt

Freshly ground black pepper

At home: Heat a large saucepan over medium heat for a few moments. Add the oil, onions, and pancetta or guanciale, if using, and cook until the onion is golden, about 5 minutes. Adjust the heat as necessary to prevent the onion from burning. Add the carrots and celery, stir well, and cook together for 5 minutes more. Add the lentils, rosemary, and bay leaf, stir, and cook for 5 minutes more. Then add enough of the stock to cover the lentils by about 1 inch.

Adjust the heat to maintain a simmer, and cook, uncovered, stirring every 10 minutes, for 25 to 35 minutes, until the lentils are soft. If the pan begins to dry out, add more stock, but be judicious about how much liquid you add. As with a risotto, you do not want any liquid left at the end.

Remove and discard the bay leaf, rosemary, and pancetta or guanciale, if using. Stir in the butter and the parsley. Taste for seasoning—unless the stock was very salty, you will need to add salt and 2 grindings of black pepper. You can store them in an airtight container in the refrigerator for up to 5 days.

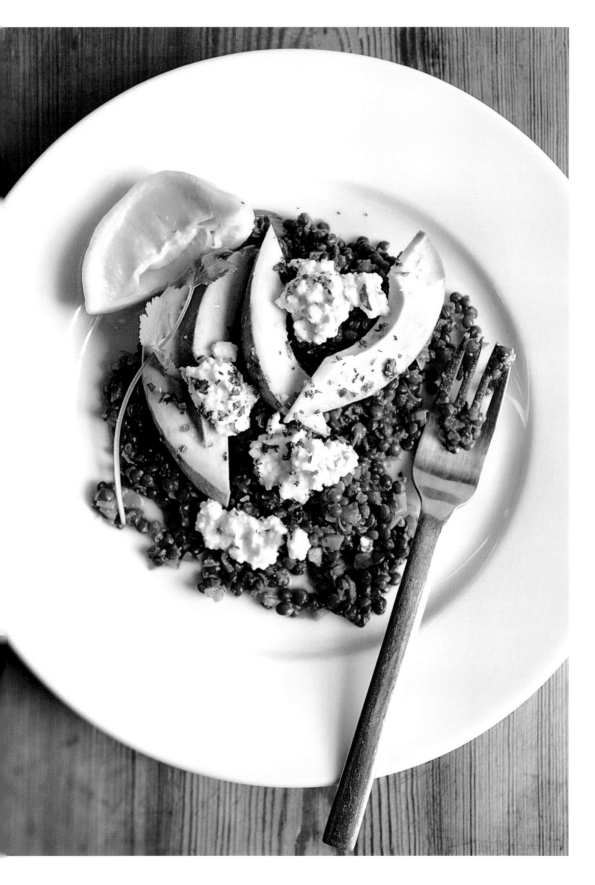

Lentils, Laid Out with Avocado and Feta

SERVES FOUR.

At the shop:

1 cup cooked lentils (see page 70)

1 ripe avocado, halved, pitted, peeled, and sliced

1 lemon

Salt

Freshly ground black pepper

½ cup cilantro and/or mint leaves, chopped

4 ounces feta cheese

2 tablespoons olive oil

So simple: a small construct of parts and textures and tastes, perfectly balanced. It is the lightness that you are after—the flavors all pleased to see one another. After making the lentils at home, the rest of this dish's preparation can take place at the shop.

At the shop: Warm the lentils, and divide them among 4 plates. Lay the avocado slices across the lentils, dividing them among the plates. Squeeze a little lemon juice over the avocado, season with a little salt and pepper, and sprinkle a good handful of the cilantro and/or mint over all of it. (Save a little of the chopped cilantro/mint to go on the feta, the next level up.)

In a small bowl, crumble the feta with a fork. Mix in the oil, a squeeze of lemon, and a pinch of the chopped herbs. Stir once or twice, very lightly, and then spoon the feta mixture equally over the four plates.

THE CORPS DE LENTILS

There is a quiet master of lentils in Seattle: Kent Stowell, former codirector, with his wife, Francia Russell, of the Pacific Northwest Ballet (PNB). They came to Seattle in 1977 after dancing for Balanchine at the New York City Ballet and then running the Frankfurt Ballet. They settled in to raise three boys and to grow the very young PNB into a remarkable ballet company and school.

Perhaps it is the influence of being the choreographer of *Swan Lake, Carmina Burana, Romeo and Juliet,* and *The Nutcracker*—whatever the case, Kent has a remarkable talent for getting six or seven or eight different parts of a wonderful meal to arrive on course and on time. And in proper line. Invariably, lentils are part of the company.

Often, he will serve lentils with sautéed greens and onions and bits of chicken or duck. He will keep a saucepan with slow-rolling stock on the back burner of his stove and use that to loosen and sustain the lentils.

Kent is the perfect example of the continuation of cooking: When he is finishing the dinner, he is already quietly choreographing the next day's lunch. The lentils will go beneath the lamb; the roasted potatoes will come in alongside them. The lentils are a crucial part of his routine. All his boys cook, but the youngest, Ethan, is a superstar chef. He has five restaurants in Seattle, and that number is likely to grow to eight or ten. And it is also likely that their menus will feature lentils, one way or another.

A Third Way to Cook Lentils

SERVES FOUR.

This method for cooking the lentils takes a bit longer and requires a little more attention. It is similar to making a bean soup and is, to my mind, the best method for precooking lentils if you are making a lentil soup.

The vegetables must cook until they sweeten, and then they must combine with the tomatoes and lentils, able to be tasted but barely in sight. The tomatoes broaden the taste of the vegetables.

At home: In a medium saucepan, heat the oil over medium heat. Add the onions and pancetta or guanciale, if using, and cook, stirring to prevent them from sticking, for 5 minutes, until lightly browned. Add the celery and carrots, stir, and then add the tomatoes (with juice). Reduce the heat to low, and cook, uncovered, stirring every 5 minutes or so, for 20 to 30 minutes. If the pan begins to look dry, add a small ladleful of stock. You are, in effect, making a tomato sauce for the lentils.

When the tomato base is well-combined, add the lentils and stir. Cook for 4 minutes, and then add enough stock to cover the lentils by about 1 inch. Bring the mixture to a slow boil and cover. Cook, stirring once or twice and checking to make sure the pan is not drying out, for 30 to 35 minutes. The lentils should be soft, and the consistency of the mixture should be thick. Taste to check the texture of the lentils, and season with salt and pepper, as needed. Remove and discard the pancetta, or guanciale, if using.

Reduce the heat to low. Process one-third of the lentils through a ricer back into the pan, and add 1 cup of the stock, stirring to combine. You may need a little more stock to reach the desired consistency, especially if you are making a soup (see Lentil Soup, Straight Up, page 74). Some like it when a wooden spoon can stand up in their soup, and some want the spoon to fall over.

Let the lentils cool. Use them immediately—for instance, you could make a simple side dish by adding a little cooked white rice and a tiny splash of red wine vinegar. Otherwise, transfer them to an airtight container and store them in the refrigerator for later use. They will keep for 5 to 7 days.

At home:

2 tablespoons olive oil

1 yellow onion, finely chopped

1 piece (3 ounces) of pancetta or guanciale (optional)

1 celery stalk, finely chopped

1 carrot, finely chopped

½ cup fresh or canned peeled tomatoes, roughly chopped (with juice)

6 to 8 cups warm chicken or vegetable stock

1 cup lentils, soaked

Salt

Freshly ground black pepper

½ cup cooked white rice

1 tablespoon red wine vinegar

Lentil Soup, Straight Up

At home:

2 cups cooked lentils (see page 73)

1 cup warm chicken or vegetable stock

4 tablespoons (½ stick) cold butter, cut into ½-inch pieces

½ cup freshly grated Parmesan cheese

Salt

Freshly ground black pepper

½ cup fresh flat-leaf parsley leaves, chopped

At the shop:

Freshly ground black pepper

½ cup freshly grated Parmesan cheese

Handful of fresh flat-leaf parsley leaves, chopped

I love lentil soup—by itself or as a remarkable base to which other ingredients can be added. There have been times in cold weather when we have had lentil soup for lunch on Monday, lentil soup with rice and chicken on Tuesday, and lentil soup with roasted potatoes and chopped ham on Wednesday. And no one has complained.

At home: In a medium saucepan, warm the lentils. Stir in the warm stock, adding more or less to obtain the desired consistency. Stir the butter pieces into the lentils, with some vigor, as you would when making a risotto. Once the butter has been fully combined, add the Parmesan and stir until it has melted into the mixture. Taste the soup, and season with salt and pepper, as needed, then stir in the parsley. Serve immediately, or let the soup cool, transfer it to an airtight container, and store it in the refrigerator. It will keep for several days.

At the shop: Reheat the soup, stirring well so that it does not stick. Grind some pepper over the top, sprinkle with Parmesan, finish with parsley, and serve.

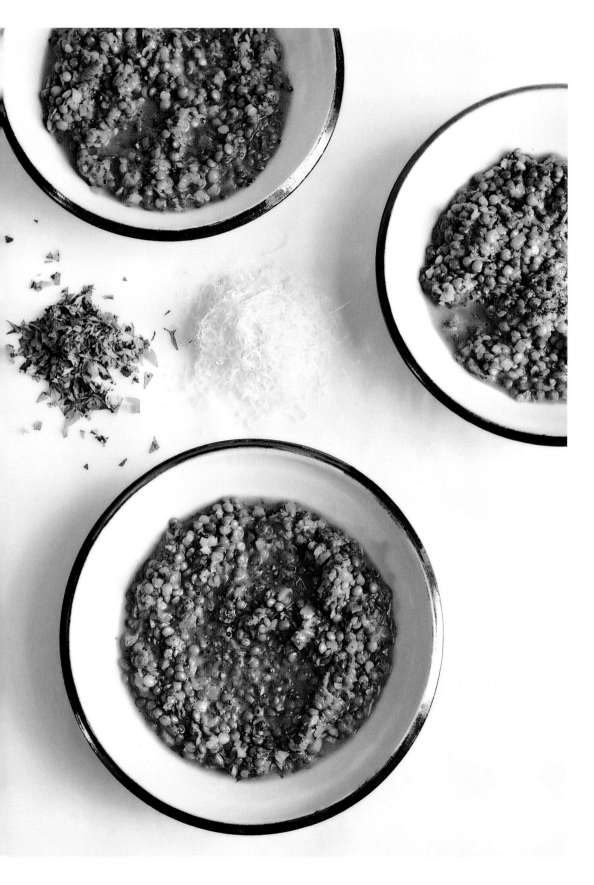

Lentils Dressed to Join a Salad

SERVES FOUR.

This is a kind of honor parade for the lentils, set amid colorful tomatoes, peppers, and feta. Taste the lentils all by themselves—they are the lead singer in this ensemble.

You can make this dish with any cooked lentils. After making them at home, the rest of this dish's preparation can take place at the shop. Romaine is a good choice for the lettuce because it holds its shape, but any variety of lettuce would work. Make sure to wash the cherry tomatoes thoroughly, as they are likely to have experienced quite a bit of handling.

At the shop: Slice the onion crosswise into six to eight ½-inch rounds and place them in a bowl. Add the vinegar, and sprinkle with salt. Set aside.

In a small bowl, add a squeeze of lemon and the mustard to the vinaigrette, and whisk with a fork to combine.

Cut a very small piece from the chili; it should be slightly hot, not blowtorch hot. If you have mistakenly purchased the blowtorch variety, carefully cut 2 tiny rounds from the chili, then cut them into even tinier pieces, and save the rest in a zip-top bag. Wash your hands *immediately* after handling the pepper, and avoid touching your eyes. If your pepper is the right mildness, cut it crosswise into thin rounds, and place them in the bowl with the onions.

Cut the tomatoes in half and salt them lightly.

Use your largest mixing bowl to assemble the salad—you want the parts to have a little room to stretch and not be clumped together. Place the greens in the bowl, add the vinaigrette, and toss to coat the leaves. Add the lentils and toss 2 or 3 times. Add the tomatoes.

Drain the onion mixture, add to the salad, and toss twice again. Sprinkle with the cheese, breaking it up against the side of the bowl with a fork. Taste for salt; the cheese, tomatoes, and lentils will all contribute a bit of salt, so you may not need to season much further.

Lay the salad on plates or pasta bowls. You want it slightly deconstructed, with onion slices poking up and bits of tomato, cheese, and chili lying about. Grind fresh pepper over each plate, and then add a squeeze of lemon and a tiny drizzle of oil. The lentils will look wonderful mixing in with all the colors, shapes, and textures.

At the shop:

1 small red onion

1 teaspoon white wine vinegar

Salt

½ lemon

½ teaspoon mustard

¼ cup A Very Good Basic Vinaigrette (see page 51)

1 long, skinny red pepper, mirasol or mild cayenne

6 to 8 cherry tomatoes

1 small head romaine or Bibb lettuce, torn into 2-inch pieces

½ cup cooked lentils (see page 67, 70, or 73)

4 ounces feta cheese

Freshly ground black pepper

2 tablespoons olive oil

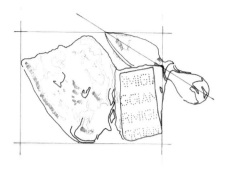

PASTA

Forty years ago in Seattle, you had to drive out near the airport to get a good plate of pasta. You never even heard the word *pasta*—only *spaghetti*. And the only basil around was dried basil in a spice jar. Parmesan came in a green cardboard cylinder.

Now they serve pasta salads on airplanes, and you can buy them to go in gas stations, and no one thinks the word *pasta* is an affectation. It has become, in a way, common, and that has lowered our expectations of it.

The true task of serving pasta for lunch is mastering the subtlety of its not appearing as a lump or sitting sullenly as a leftover—and not tasting like a lump or a leftover. When you are making pasta at home, there is an immediacy to the meal—the pasta goes from pot to table. But the next day is a different matter, and certain details can make an enormous difference. The shape of the pasta, for example, will dictate what you can and cannot do. Very wide pappardelle pasta can be quite wonderful when served with the lightest butter and sage sauce, but by the next day, the pappardelle has gained weight and lost some gentleness and must be handled quite differently. You can warm it for two minutes in a microwave or, if you have a burner, slightly sauté it in a little heated water. After warming it, cut the pappardelle into three-inch lengths; this will lighten its effect.

Similarly, penne, which stores much of the sauce in its grooves and tubing, can appear quite inert the next day coming out of the refrigerator. You must take steps to bring it back to life. Let the pasta come at least close to room temperature. If you are using it for a salad, put it into the microwave for fifteen to twenty seconds to loosen it. If it is being fully reheated as a pasta, add half a glass of heated water and stir vigorously to incorporate it into the pasta before putting the dish into the microwave.

You must know what is in the pasta before serving it at lunch. If it has seafood in it, omit Parmesan and add lemon juice, olive oil, and chopped parsley to bring back the dish's youth. If it is a cream sauce, then pause the reheating after a minute to stir and mix. If it is a tomato base, adding a little water or even a pat of butter during reheating will smooth the texture. If there is a great deal of cheese or sugar in the sauce, then you must take extra precaution that it does not burn on the bottom; either pause the microwave halfway through and stir, or stay by the pan and stir as it warms.

Pasta made at home often makes the base for a future lunch. It may be that I accidentally cook a bit more than needed for a meal. Or the pasta water is still simmering, and bits of leftovers from dinner are still on the counter—a little parsley, some Parmesan, a few peas, half a tomato, some bread crumbs. Keeping the next day's lunch in mind, I will toss a handful of spaghetti into the pasta water while I clean up. When the pasta is done, I drain it and pour it into a mixing bowl, then add some olive oil or a pat of butter, some salt, and all the bits and leftovers—even carrots or a sprig of rosemary or the juice of half a lemon or the meat of a chicken leg. I taste, grind some fresh pepper, and add a little reserved pasta water if the mixture is dry; then I'm ready for tomorrow's lunch. If you try the same approach, you will be surprised and, I hope, amused at how you have cleaned your kitchen and at the same time prepared lunch.

The pasta may be a meal of its own, or act as a side to a salad, or add character to a soup. I have stared glumly at a cold plate of leftover penne, my only partner for a lunch. But find a creamy soup or a cup of hot chili to fold into the pasta; add, perhaps, a little feta, parsley, and a bit of lemon; and your spirits may well rejoin you.

If your pasta is to be fully reheated, be certain to heat the plates as well: It is a shame to put warm pasta on a cold plate.

Finally, if you are making pasta specifically for lunch, it is best to keep it simple . . .

PASTA AT CAPE BRETON

My first leftover pasta lunch was eaten in Nova Scotia, oddly enough. Having finished graduate school in Boston, I headed north to do some hiking and exploring in Maine for the summer. The farther north I traveled, the more I heard about Nova Scotia. I decided to take a look.

It was easy enough to hitchhike in Maine, but the rides grew scarce in Newfoundland. I was about to turn back, when I met up with Dino, a graduate student from NYU, and his girlfriend, Sarah, as they were getting gas at a rest stop. They graciously took me with them to Cape Breton, where they had rented a fishing cabin on a steep hillside in a coastal town called Meat Cove. We could see icebergs and whales from the front deck, and catch lobster by hand, and I had my first and only wild strawberry pie, for there were enough wild strawberries.

Dino's mom came up from Brooklyn to visit. She had no more interest in Nova Scotia than in cedar stumps, but she loved Dino. During the visit, she made an enormous pot of spaghetti and meat sauce for dinner (no one said "Bolognese"; it was 1968). The next day, Dino and I were trudging up from the beach to the cabin high above, a steep hike, and he laughed and said, "Leftover pasta for lunch!" He heated a pan on the electric stove, added some olive oil, then the pasta, then a bit of warmed water, and stirred until it was just heated through. I had never seen spaghetti in a frying pan. And I never forgot that plate of pasta.

Pasta with Your Tomato Sauce, Made to Order

SERVES FOUR.

At home:

Salt

¼ cup olive oil

2 garlic cloves, finely chopped

1 can (28 ounces) peeled San Marzano plum tomatoes with juice

½ cup fresh basil leaves

Freshly ground black pepper

1 pound pasta (spaghetti, linguine, penne, or rigatoni)

½ cup freshly grated Parmesan cheese

At the shop:

½ cup freshly grated Parmesan cheese

½ cup fresh basil leaves

There are many recipes for pasta with tomato sauce—this is one. Tomatoes and garlic, basil and olive oil, salt and pepper, pasta and Parmesan: If you use the best quality of each of them, then this is a brilliant pasta.

Instead of cooking and serving pasta with the sauce, you could save the tomato sauce for other uses. Stored in a tightly sealed jar, it will keep in the refrigerator for a week. Heated separately, you can pour it over any cooked pasta, chicken, sausage, or meat loaf.

At home: Bring a large pot of salted water to a boil.

In a saucepan, warm the oil over medium heat for a moment. Quickly add the garlic, tomatoes with juice (smash them beforehand, through your fingers or with a slotted spoon), and basil, and stir to combine. Add 1 teaspoon of salt and a couple grinds of pepper, stir again, and simmer, uncovered, for 25 minutes.

When the sauce has been cooking for about 15 minutes, add the pasta to the boiling water, and stir to prevent clumping. Boil the pasta for about 10 minutes, then check to see if it is ready. If not, continue to cook for 1 to 2 minutes more, then check again.

Pour 1 cup of the boiling pasta-cooking water into a large ceramic or stainless-steel serving bowl to heat the bowl, and let sit for 3 minutes. Pour the water out. Drain the pasta and quickly transfer it to the heated bowl. Top the cooked pasta with half of the Parmesan, and pour half of the tomato sauce into the bowl. Toss quickly, then add a little salt and half of the remaining sauce and toss again. Finally, top with the remaining sauce and some pepper.

Transfer the cooked pasta to an airtight container and refrigerate.

At the shop: Add 2 tablespoons of water at the start to loosen the pasta sauce. Reheat the pasta either in the microwave (for about 2 to 3 minutes) or in a sauté pan over a burner (for about 5 minutes). When the pasta is hot, add the Parmesan and stir it well, so that it melts. Add the basil right before serving.

Linguine with Pancetta, Basil, and Cherry Tomatoes

SERVES FOUR.

A very workaday pasta—you can even make it as you are washing the dishes from dinner.

At home: Bring a large pot of salted water to a boil.

In a medium sauté pan, heat the oil over medium heat. Add the garlic and sauté until it begins to color but not burn. Remove and discard the garlic. Add the pancetta and the red pepper and stir to coat them in the oil. Add a grind of black pepper, and cook for 3 to 4 minutes, until the pancetta begins to crisp.

Add the linguine or spaghetti to the pot of boiling water and cook until al dente, following the guidelines on the package. (As you learn this dish, you will have the pasta cooking even before the pancetta has crisped.)

Rinse the tomatoes and add them, still wet, to the pan with the pancetta. Cook, stirring, for no more than 1 minute.

Drain the pasta, reserving ½ cup of the cooking water, and then quickly add the cooked linguine to the pan with the tomatoes and pancetta. Stir to coat, season with a little salt, and quickly stir in the butter. Add the basil and fold into the pasta. If the mixture is too dry, very quickly add some of the reserved cooking water and toss.

The pasta will keep in an airtight container in the refrigerator for 3 to 4 days.

At the shop: Reheat the pasta until it is quite hot. Sprinkle some of the Parmesan on top, then taste and season with salt and pepper, as needed. Just before serving, drizzle the pasta with a little olive oil. Use forks to serve the pasta, so it will sit loose and slightly separated on the plate. The last ingredients have a much greater effect if added fresh at the very end, rather than at home.

Variation: This dish would also be a wonderful pasta salad, in which case, reheat the pasta for just a moment. Add 4 or 5 fresh cherry tomatoes, halved and salted, just before serving.

At home:

Salt

¼ cup olive oil

1 garlic clove

¼ pound pancetta, cut into strips

1 dried hot red pepper

Freshly ground black pepper

1 pound linguine or spaghetti

12 cherry tomatoes

1 tablespoon cold butter

12 to 16 small basil leaves

At the shop:

½ cup freshly grated Parmesan cheese

Salt

Freshly ground black pepper

Olive oil

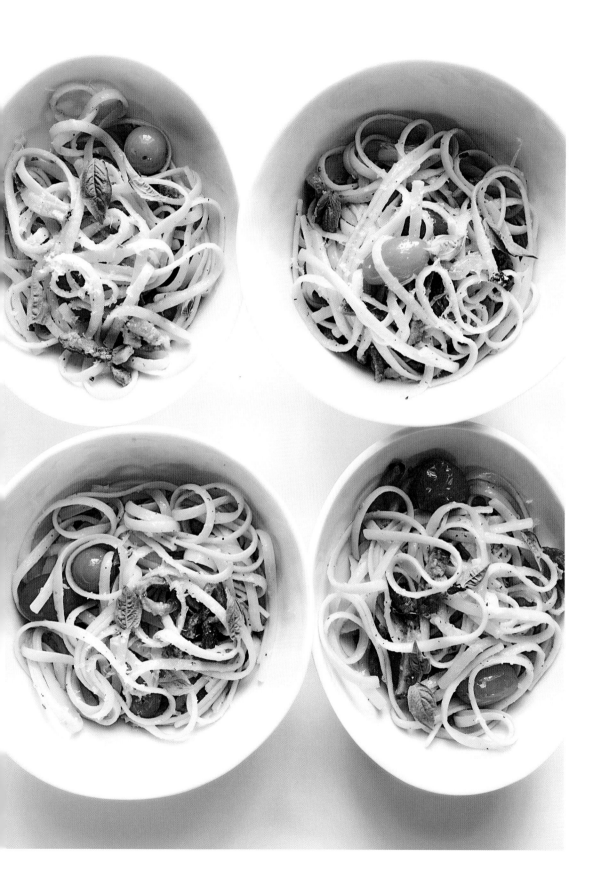

A Salad for Pasta with Tomato Sauce

SERVES FOUR.

Any pasta, plain or sauced, may also be wonderful later in a salad, especially if it is not too saucy or creamy. It is a revival: The pasta is not going to show much life until you set a stage and make some arrangements. For this, there are a few tips that can be helpful. Use less of the pasta than you might imagine. And let it come to room temperature. Mix the greens first, on their own, so their dressing and seasoning is correct, and arrange them on the plates. Then toss the pasta in the empty salad bowl to collect what dressing is left. Use a very light dressing, so you do not add too much weight to the already dense pasta.

Once the pasta is in the bowl, you might add olives, chives, scallions, cherry tomatoes, a spoonful of yogurt, or a quick crumble of feta. Top each plate of greens with a spoonful of the pasta salad. To finish, add sesame seeds or parsley and, if need be, lemon juice. If you have any fruit or tangy pickled onions, plate them to the side of the salad.

One of my favorite pasta salads is this one—made of a leftover pasta with tomato sauce, a common inhabitant in my fridge. Any pasta with a tomato sauce (whether the one on page 79 or another version) already has some heft, so pair it with prickly or skinny greens—arugula, mâche, parsley, cilantro, or dandelion. And make the dressing skinny, as well. Remember to always use slightly less pasta than you think you'll need when making a salad—you can always add a bit more. The lemon and cracked pepper serve to keep the parts from gumming together.

At the shop: In a serving bowl, combine the vinegar and a good pinch of salt, and let the salt dissolve. With a fork, stir in the oil. Crack some pepper and squeeze half of the lemon into the dressing. Stir well to emulsify; the dressing should be quite liquid from the lemon.

Add the greens and half of the parsley and cilantro, and mix them very quickly in the dressing. Quickly divide the dressed greens among 4 large plates. Sprinkle the feta lightly over the greens.

Put the pasta into the salad bowl with the leftover dressing and toss it, separating the pasta strands with a fork. Divide the pasta among the plates, laying it gently on top of the greens. Sprinkle with the remaining parsley and cilantro, and drizzle with juice from the remaining ½ lemon. Add 2 good cracks of pepper and a little salt, and the dish is ready.

At the shop:

1 tablespoon red wine vinegar

Salt

¼ cup olive oil

Freshly ground black pepper

1 lemon

2 cups mixed greens (only the skinny and spicy varieties will work)

¼ cup fresh flat-leaf parsley leaves, chopped

¼ cup fresh cilantro leaves, chopped

2 tablespoons crumbled feta cheese

1 cup leftover Pasta with Your Tomato Sauce, Made to Order (see page 79), or similar recipe

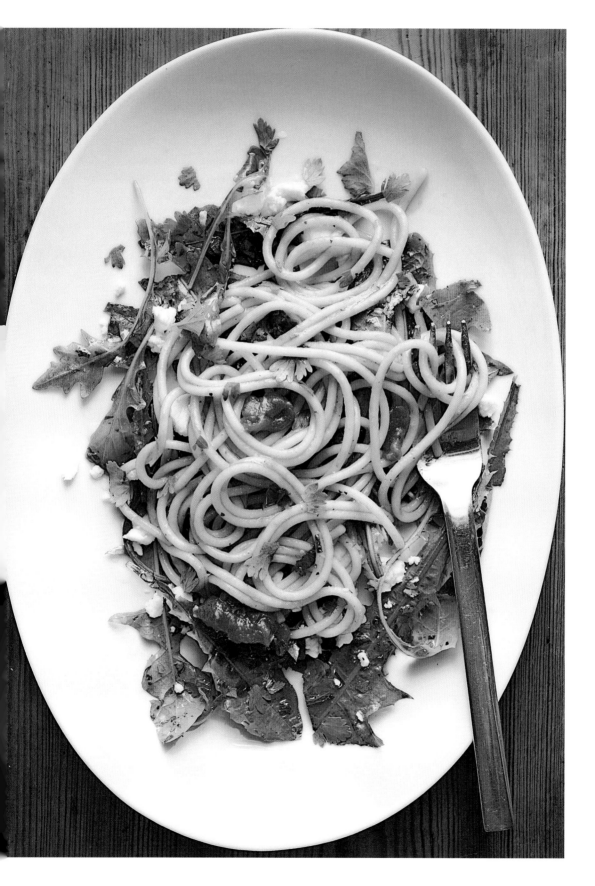

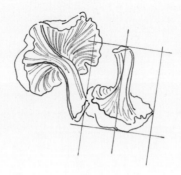

RICE

We use rice so often that it is easily taken for granted. Any leftover rice is tossed into whatever soup is going, or any salad after it is dressed. In winter, we make rice with peas and sausages at home, and I always make extra, for it is wonderful the next day. By spring, the first local asparagus and Walla Walla onions become a risotto base. During summer or fall, we add chanterelle mushrooms, some chopped and stirred in at the start, and some, barely cooked, laid atop the risotto.

One of our favorite ways to prepare rice, risotto is a wealth not of material but of detail and technique and attention. You can make the very same risotto fifty times, and each time it will be slightly different. And the more times you make the risotto, the more you will notice the differences.

Rice dishes reheat quite well the next day, but keep the portions small, for they are rich and filling. You must be certain to make a very simple salad to go with these dishes, or a relish, such as a mango chutney or a pickled plum—something to add sparkle to the rice.

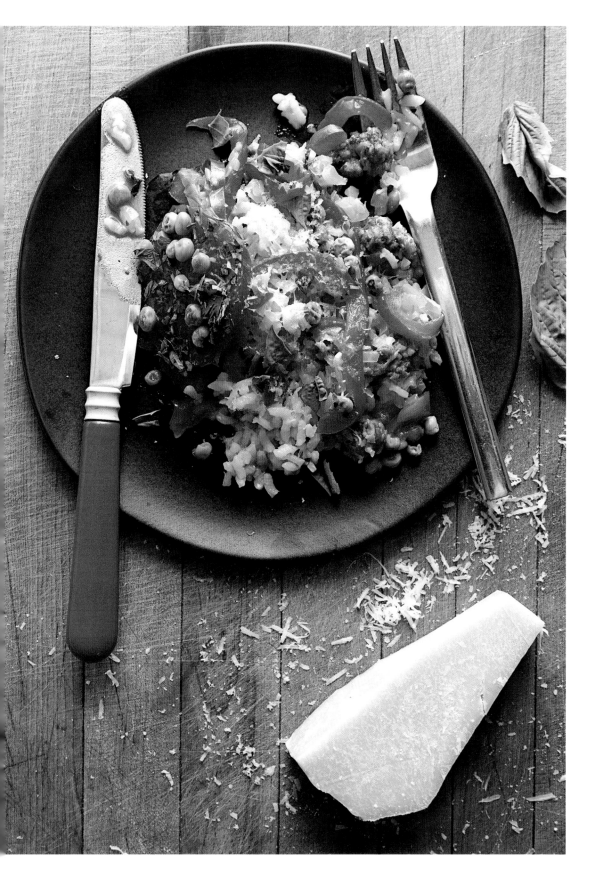

A Spanish Rice with Sausage and Peas

SERVES FOUR.

Keep this recipe in mind. It can be a great help at dinner—much of the work is done in the oven. You will need a heavy cast-iron pan with a good lid for this (a 5-quart round enameled Le Creuset is ideal). Once you have assembled the ingredients in the cast-iron pan and put the lid on, you are free to work on other parts of the meal. The recipe is also a fine example of the importance of layering ingredients and timing. And it is perfectly suited to being served for lunch the next day.

It begins like a risotto, with sautéing the onions, toasting the rice, adding a bit of wine or sherry. But then it goes in its own direction.

At home: Preheat the oven to 375°F.

Heat a cast-iron pan over medium heat. Add the oil and butter, and once the butter has melted, add the onions and cook for 5 minutes. Add the red peppers and the sausage and cook, breaking up the sausage with a wooden spoon and stirring well to keep the onions from sticking, for 5 minutes.

Add the garlic, stir, and cook for 2 minutes. Add the rice, stir to coat, and cook for 2 to 3 minutes to barely toast the rice. Add the wine; it should sizzle for a moment when it hits the pan. Stir it well to combine and then cook for 1 to 2 minutes until it has evaporated.

Add the stock. The liquid should cover the rice by no more than 1 inch. Stir one last time to make certain nothing is sticking to the bottom of the pan and to ensure that the ingredients are well-combined. Cover the pan and carefully place it in the oven.

Bake the rice for 25 minutes. Carefully remove it from the oven. Uncover the pan, lay the tomato slices and the peas on the surface, and quickly put the lid back on. (Keeping the heat in will steam the peas and the tomatoes.) Chop the basil and parsley together. After 10 minutes, uncover the pan and add the basil and parsley, stirring them carefully into the dish. Taste and season with salt and pepper. Add a little grated Parmesan while the rice is hot, sprinkling it on top. Serve immediately, or let the rice cool to room temperature, transfer it to an airtight container, and refrigerate it.

At the shop: Reheat the rice in the microwave, or sauté it in oil for a couple of minutes, with a splash of warmed water added for either method. Add the Parmesan and parsley just before serving.

At home:

¼ cup olive oil

4 tablespoons good butter

1 yellow or Spanish onion, finely chopped

1 red bell pepper, seeded and cut into strips

1 hot Italian sausage, casing removed

1 garlic clove, finely chopped

1 cup Carnaroli rice

¼ cup white wine or sherry

3 cups slowly boiling chicken or vegetable stock

2 tomatoes, sliced

¾ cup fresh or thawed frozen peas

12 fresh basil leaves, roughly shredded

¼ cup fresh flat-leaf parsley leaves, roughly shredded

Salt

Freshly ground black pepper

¼ cup freshly grated Parmesan cheese

At the shop:

¼ cup olive oil (optional)

¼ cup freshly grated Parmesan cheese

¼ cup fresh flat-leaf parsley leaves, chopped

Variations: Saffron: You can, of course, omit the sausage, switch the stock to a non-meat variety, and make a vegetarian rice. If you do, consider adding 1 teaspoon of saffron (soaked first in 2 tablespoons warm stock), just after adding the wine, to bring saffron's lovely yellow color and signature taste to the dish.

Asparagus: In the spring, blanch some trimmed fresh asparagus (8 to 10 stalks) in boiling salted water for 2 minutes. Remove the tips from the stems and then chop the stems into 2-inch lengths. (Save the tips to add at the end with the tomatoes and peas.) Add the asparagus stem pieces to the rice just before it goes into the oven.

EAT YOUR PEAS

Poor peas. Sixty years ago, the best plea that parents could make was "Eat your peas!" and in our family, at least, many of them ended up behind the radiator. They had come from a can or, if they were fresh, they were overcooked, and both methods left them sour. Children are very quick to sense and veer from sour.

But we have escaped from the cooking of the Cold War, and peas have survived that terrible format. They can now be what they had always claimed—sweet and wonderful. The process of freezing them is quite subtle and if you let them first thaw a bit and then quickly boil them in salted water, they can be wonderful. The caution is that you not overcook them. Also, frozen peas of a good and recent quality will retain their vivid green color better even than fresh peas.

But keep an eye out for fresh peas as well. They begin to arrive in the spring. In Seattle, they are near full strength by the middle of July; the pods are plump with peas trying to get out. Even our cat loves them. She will race to the kitchen at the sound of pods being opened, corral the ones that have dropped, and eat at once.

They are fine eaten raw in salads or even in a bowl with some pecorino cheese. If you are careful not to overcook them, you can literally add fresh peas to every dish you will serve—and none will be abandoned behind the radiator.

A Basic Risotto

SERVES THREE TO FOUR.

At home:

5 tablespoons cold unsalted butter

I onion, finely chopped

2 cups Carnaroli rice

½ cup dry white wine

7 cups hot chicken or vegetable stock

I cup freshly grated Parmesan cheese

Salt

Freshly ground black pepper

I tablespoon fresh flat-leaf parsley leaves, chopped

At the shop:

½ cup freshly grated Parmesan cheese

Salt

Freshly ground black pepper

Risotto is a specific place between too much and too little heat. It is a brisk pace, neither a run nor a stroll. You must find the right temperature for your stove top and your pans. Too low, and you will be dragging the risotto uphill; too high, and you will be chasing it downhill. There is a common saying about risotto: Never make it unless you are in a good mood.

No matter how good your humor, you also need the right pan to make risotto. It must be a heavy-bottomed saucepan, not too big and not too narrow, and it must have a good handle that you can hold while the pan is over eager heat. You must stir for twenty minutes, and then stir again, more vigorously, when you add the butter and cheese. There are a few other essentials: wooden spoons only; good stock, kept at a simmer; onions chopped smaller than the grains of rice; grated Parmesan; cold, cold butter; white wine; and Carnaroli rice. The Carnaroli rice will help add a wonderful creaminess to it all.

Should you have leftover peas, carrots, or root vegetables, heat them and fold them into the risotto just before serving. Or on lucky days when you have a bit of beef stew or Bolognese sauce left, heat it separately and serve it over the heated risotto. Top the dish with Parmesan—an enviable lunch, especially in the cold months. See the variations for more of our favorite ideas.

At home: In a large, heavy-bottomed saucepan, melt 1 tablespoon of the butter over medium heat. Add the onions and cook, stirring, for 2 minutes (this will get you and the onion warmed up). Cook until the onion is translucent but not browned. Add the rice and stir to coat, then cook, stirring, for 2 to 3 minutes, to toast the rice in the butter. Add the white wine; it should sizzle a little and then simmer. If it does not sizzle, the temperature of the pan is too low; if it evaporates away immediately, the pan is too hot. Cook for 1 to 2 minutes, until the liquid has evaporated.

Add a ladleful of stock—again, it should sizzle a bit. Now the risotto has begun its 18- to 20-minute journey to completion. Cook, stirring, until the rice has almost completely absorbed the stock. Repeat 12 to 14 more times, adding stock and stirring until it has been absorbed. This is not the time to take a phone call, and you will not be the first person to wish for a machine to do the stirring, or at least a gullible nephew. Scrape the sides, stir to the middle, add the stock—after 12 minutes or so, you will feel the difference in your wooden spoon: the rice slightly expanding, slightly softening, its starches smoothing the sauce.

As the risotto cooks, absorbing more and more stock, it will expand, and you will need to hold the handle tightly to stir. The pan will be heavy, but your stirring must be vigorous, lifting the bottom and the sides and the belly of the risotto so it cooks evenly, stays on the heat, and keeps pushing itself.

After 18 to 20 minutes, taste the risotto; it is done when the rice is cooked but still has a slight al dente firmness to it. You should still have a little stock left. If the risotto is too thick, stir in the final bit of liquid to loosen it.

Take the pan off the heat, cover it, and let it stand for 1 minute. Uncover the pan and stir in the remaining 4 tablespoons of butter; stir it with force, getting the butter to melt into it all. Add ½ cup of the Parmesan, stir well, and then taste the risotto. It may need salt, but it may not. The stock, cheese, and butter will all lend a degree of saltiness to the dish.

Add one quick grind of pepper, and then serve the risotto in heated wide bowls (do not complete all this work and then use cold dishes!), dusted with some of the remaining cheese and the parsley.

At the shop: Risotto is a dish so intimate with timing that it will not be the same the day after it is made, but it can still be wonderful. Stir in ½ cup of warmed water and reheat the risotto in the microwave, pausing the microwave frequently to stir. Once hot (make sure it is hot, not simply lukewarm), divide the risotto among warmed plates, and top with the Parmesan and a touch of salt and pepper.

Variations: Prosciutto. Once you have the risotto at the shop, there are some very simple foods that you might add or toss onto it. You might, for example, buy a very slight ¼ pound of prosciutto, thinly sliced. Roll each slice loosely up like a rug and cut each roll into thin strips. You might have to shake them a little to separate. Then toss the strips on the risotto when it is heating up, about halfway through, and add the Parmesan at the end. The prosciutto will look like a jumble of threads on top and add a wonderful salty taste.

Pistachios and parsley. You can also buy a small bag of pistachio nuts and some parsley. Shell the pistachios, add them to about ½ cup parsley leaves, and roughly chop them together. Sprinkle the mix onto the risotto just when it is fully warmed.

Chili. One cold winter lunch, we purchased a single cup of a very spicy chili, and after heating it up alongside the risotto, we poured it over the top. It was just the extra heat we needed, and the two foods worked together like old friends.

———

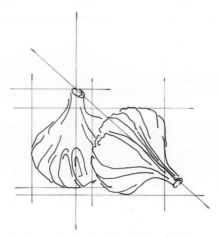

THE MEATS AND THE FISHES

Many meat and fish dishes made at home will work wonderfully for lunch and will clog up neither your time nor your kitchen.

You can, of course, simply make extra portions of whatever you are preparing for your dinner and bring those to work. Or you can cook to the side, using part of your oven or burners specifically for a next-day meal. The oven is already hot, the pans are out, the cutting boards are half-empty—a perfect time to prep. Roasting a piece of chicken or a beef cut or a fish fillet can all be done quite easily while you have the kitchen running and the leftover ingredients from dinner lying about.

Once you have cooked the meat or the piece of fish, it is an easy task to pair it the next day with a salad or a little pasta or to fold it into pita bread as an informal sandwich. Keep in mind texture and heartiness and subtlety: A tenderloin can match with anything from sweet plums to horseradish, but a piece of salmon has quieter allies. If you are uncertain, proceed slowly. Start with a little lemon juice and try a small bite. Or lay out a couple of options in small bowls—a green sauce or a salsa, a mustard, and a mayonnaise; pickles and olives; hummus and yogurt—and then let each person dabble for themselves.

At the shop, fuss for a moment. Choose a plate that you like, add a bit of fresh chopped parsley, sprinkle a little salt, and grind some pepper, even if just to the side. (Your store-bought roast beef sandwich may come with a sprig of parsley, but you can do much better than that!) Quarter a lemon, add a few pieces of marinated onions, cut a pickle into smaller slivers. Your greatest task is presentation, and you have an arsenal of ingredients at your disposal.

When you are bringing in leftover meats from home, instead of just making a sandwich with sliced breads, also try the smaller rolls. Then you can make each one slightly different—one with chutney, one with mustard and ketchup, one with horse-radish and mayonnaise. On the smaller stage of a roll, you can experiment—and use up any good bits and pieces that may have ended up in your fridge. And always check if you have any greens that need to be put to work. They may need to be chopped or dressed in a vinaigrette, but even a small amount of greens are good company for meat and fish.

Ways to Bring a Chicken to Lunch

I remember grumbling when someone brought a supermarket-roasted, boneless, skinless chicken breast to lunch. I argued that you have no way to tell how fresh it is or how fresh it was, no sense of how it was seasoned or handled—its only virtue is convenience. But mostly I argued that a single chicken breast is so easily done at home, and done well, that you should make the effort.

The simplest way, of course, is to salt and pepper the breast, rub it with olive oil, sprinkle a little rosemary on it, if you have some, and roast it in a low-sided roasting pan, pie tin, or frying pan in a 400°F oven for 25 minutes, turning it after the first 10 minutes. When it is done, let it cool, add a little more salt, and wrap it up for lunch the next day. Simple enough, and it will be better than any convenient chicken breast you can find, especially if it was fresh when you bought it. If possible, choose a chicken breast that is still on the bone. Prepare it the same way, but tuck some seasoning under the skin and roast it for 45 minutes, turning after 20 minutes. The bone will protect and keep the meat more moist. Once the breast has cooled, it is quite easy to lift the bone away.

In the following pages, there are two slightly more involved recipes for cooking chicken breasts; they are both favorites. Cooking a chicken breast well does have its tricks and subtleties—intimate details such as freshness, chill, oven temperature, dampness, pan size, and weight will be crucial to the results. Buy good, fresh chickens, do not crowd the pan, and always get the oven hot.

Garlic and Rosemary Chicken Breasts

SERVES TWO TO FOUR.

At home:

2 chicken breasts, skin on, bone in (not more than ¾ pound each)

1 sprig fresh rosemary

Salt

1 garlic clove, sliced very thin

¼ cup olive oil

Freshly ground black pepper

¼ cup white wine

¼ cup chicken stock

I watched three Italian grandmothers make this dish one Sunday morning in preparation for thirty guests arriving that afternoon. One did the salt, one the garlic, and one the rosemary, passing each roasting pan of chicken to the next station. They used all of the chicken—the wings and thighs and legs as well as the breasts—and, of course, you can, too.

Should you want to use a whole chicken, have it cut into parts and simply chop more rosemary and garlic, but otherwise prepare it the same way as described below. If you want to cook them all together, use a roasting pan. The pieces need enough room in the pan to caramelize a little—if they are too crowded, they will steam and stew and not form crisp edges.

If you prefer to cook just the breast, a chicken breast on the bone will indeed take a little longer to cook than its boneless cousin, but it is likely fresher (bonelessness is the last port of call). And, like a carrot with its greens, the skin and bone give the breast some defense against sitting around.

If you want to roast some vegetables, throw a few carrots, onions, slices of potato, or whatever you have on hand into the pan. It is easy to do, and they will be a welcome addition at lunch.

At home: Preheat the oven to 400°F.

Dry the chicken breasts with a paper towel. With a sharp knife, cut the chicken breasts crosswise into 4 pieces (see *Note*). You are going through some bone and the skin, so use a sharp knife, and make certain the cutting board is firm. Leave the skin attached. Wipe the pieces again with a new paper towel, feeling for any loose fragments of grit or bone.

Pull the leaves off the rosemary sprig and roughly chop them. Pour a small pile of the salt next to them. Now, carefully lift the skin from the pieces of chicken and put a good pinch of salt beneath it. Then place a couple slices of garlic beneath the skin, and finally a good pinch of the chopped rosemary.

Be careful to keep the skin attached to each piece. Drizzle oil onto the pieces and spread it over the skin with your fingers. Sprinkle the skin all over with salt, pepper, and some rosemary, especially on the underside.

Heat a sauté pan over medium for 1 minute, then add a little oil to the pan. Lay the chicken breast pieces in the pan, skin-side down, then transfer the pan to the oven.

Roast the chicken pieces for 20 minutes, then turn the pieces so they are skin-side up. They may stick a little, so use a thin spatula to loosen them and turn them, and be careful to not tear the skin.

Continue roasting the chicken for 20 minutes more. Keep an eye on the pieces: The edges where the bone and skin touch the pan should caramelize a bit, and the pan's surface will begin to brown when they are done.

Transfer the chicken pieces to a wire rack to cool—it will help to make them crispier. Set the pan over low heat, and add the white wine and stock to deglaze the pan. Scrape up any bits on the sides and bottom of the pan and let the liquids simmer for 10 minutes, adding more liquid if the pan starts to look dry. If not serving immediately, transfer the gravy to an airtight container. It can be reheated the next day and served with the chicken.

The pieces are enough for a light lunch for four, and we often serve them alongside green salads.

Note: You could leave the breasts whole, but we cut them so the pieces are of equal size and so that each browns and crisps on its own. If you leave them whole, you will get more tender white meat that can be easily sliced, but you lose some of the crispness.

———————

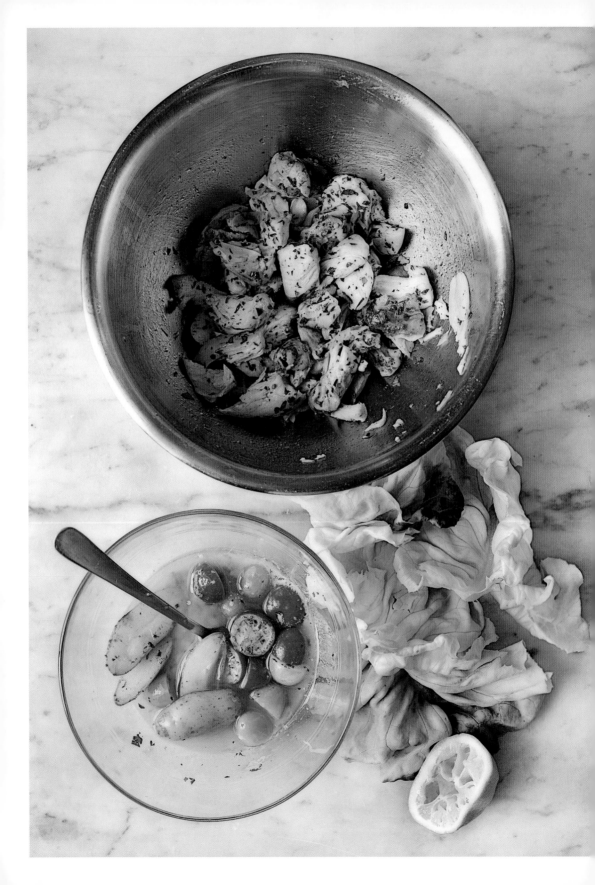

Oven-Roasted Chicken Breasts and Bibb Lettuce Salad

————————

SERVES FOUR.

You can use either the simplest way (see page 91) or the method on page 92 to roast the chicken. If you roasted a piece on the bone, be careful to remove any fragments of bone or cartilage, and use any reserved drips of gravy to flavor the dressing. This is also a fine recipe for leftover pieces of chicken from a barbecue; the combination of parsley, lemon, vinegar, and yogurt makes it all taste fresh.

At the shop: If the chicken is on the bone, remove it with your fingers, tear the flesh into smaller pieces, and put them into a bowl. Add the lemon juice, one teaspoon of the oil, the red-pepper flakes, half of the parsley, and salt and black pepper, to taste. If you are using gravy left over from roasting the chicken, loosen it with a drop or two of water and drizzle that across the pieces. Toss to combine, and set aside.

Put the vinegar in a serving bowl and add 1 teaspoon of salt and the garlic. With a fork, stir in the remaining oil until it's emulsified, add a drop or two of water, stir again, and grind some pepper on the top. Tear the lettuce leaves into palm-size pieces or smaller, and add them to the salad bowl, tossing them a couple of times to coat them in the dressing. Add the yogurt to the bowl and toss again to smear it lightly into the mix. Add the tomatoes, toss, and divide the salad among four plates.

If you have any leftover roasted potatoes or vegetables from dinner, roll them in the dressing left in the empty salad bowl, and add them to each plate alongside the salad. Gently spoon the chicken pieces over the greens, sprinkle with the remaining parsley, and top with a grind of black pepper to finish.

————————

At the shop:

2 roasted chicken breasts, at room temperature (see pages 91–93)

Juice of 1 lemon

¼ cup olive oil

Pinch of red-pepper flakes

½ cup fresh flat-leaf parsley leaves, chopped

Salt

Freshly ground black pepper

¼ to ½ cup gravy, reserved from the roasted chicken (optional)

1 tablespoon white wine vinegar

1 garlic clove, finely chopped

1 head Bibb lettuce

1 tablespoon Greek yogurt

6 to 8 cherry tomatoes, halved and lightly salted

6 to 8 roasted new red potatoes, roasted carrots, and/or onions (optional)

Breaded Boneless Chicken, in the Oven

SERVES TWO TO FOUR.

This is a very quick recipe and a great favorite, but be careful: Your fellow eaters will be spoiled when you cook this perfectly, and they will grumble when you do it poorly. Good bread crumbs are very important. Also, smaller chicken breasts will taste much better than larger ones. If we have any leftover risotto (see page 88), we often warm it up and plate this chicken over it, with a squeeze of lemon and some Parmesan. Or it makes a lovely topping for a salad.

At home: Preheat the oven to 400°F.

Check the chicken breasts for grit and bone, and dry them well with paper towels. Place the breasts in a stainless-steel bowl and add plenty of salt and pepper, then the bread crumbs. Toss to coat the chicken. Push the breasts into the crumbs that loosen, on all sides. Let stand in the bowl while you get the sauté pan ready.

Heat an ovenproof sauté pan over medium-high heat for a minute or two. Add the oil and, moments later, the butter, and melt the butter until it foams. It should sizzle but not burn or scorch. When the foam slows, add the chicken breasts—they should sizzle when they hit the pan. Cook the chicken for 2 minutes on one side to brown it, flip each breast, then cook the other side for 2 minutes more. Transfer the pan to the oven.

After 5 minutes, open the oven and flip the breasts. Cook for 4 minutes more, then carefully remove the pan from the oven; it will be hot. Let it rest for a couple of minutes. Transfer the chicken to a warm plate to rest. Set the pan over low heat (be careful, as the handle is hot—wrap it in a dishtowel, if necessary), and deglaze it with a little white wine and a sprinkling of warmed water, scraping up the browned bits from the bottom of the pan. If serving immediately, pour the sauce over the chicken and top with the parsley.

If you are cooking this for lunch, let the chicken breasts cool, then transfer them to a glass dish with an airtight lid and pour the sauce over them.

At the shop: Slice the chicken on a diagonal, across the grain, cutting toward the narrow end of the breast. Top with the parsley.

At home:

2 boneless, skinless chicken breasts, about ½ pound each

Salt

Freshly ground black pepper

1 cup bread crumbs (see page 143)

2 tablespoons olive oil

4 tablespoons unsalted butter

1 tablespoon white wine

At the shop:

¼ cup fresh flat-leaf parsley leaves, finely chopped

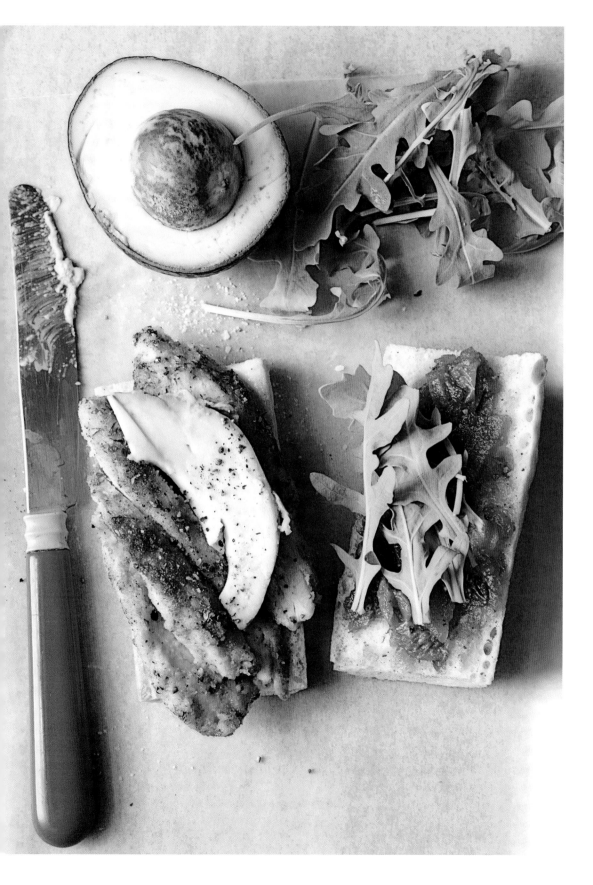

Breaded Chicken Breast Sandwich with Some Helpers

SERVES TWO TO FOUR.

It is a simple sandwich to make, and quietly popular. The small pieces of chicken are tender and a little crunchy from the breading. The chutney brings a sweet taste from underneath. The lemon and the fresh pepper keep it all sprightly. Serve the sandwiches as soon as they are assembled, for they rely on a certain freshness and on the parts remaining slightly separate.

At the shop: Bring the chicken out of the refrigerator and let it warm up on the counter.

Cut the bread or the rolls in half, on the horizontal, and lay them out like open books so you can work on them. Cut the lemon open and squeeze it on one half of each sandwich. On the other side, spread the chutney to lightly cover the surface.

Peel and slice open the avocado, remove the pit, and lay the two sections on a plate. Cut them into slices. Then sprinkle some salt and some chopped parsley or cilantro over the slices and add a good squeeze of the lemon.

The breaded chicken is best cut on a diagonal and across its grain, which runs the length of the breasts. You should get four or five pieces from each breast. Portion them out on the lemon side of each sandwich, and spoon any of the sauce directly onto the pieces. Using a tablespoon, put two or three slices of the avocado on top the chicken and the sauce.

Take a handful of the arugula and lay it on the chutney side of the sandwich; the condiment will help hold the greens in place. Tip the plate that held the avocado slices over each sandwich to let the lemon juice run off on the greens, add a pinch of salt and some fresh ground pepper, and fold the two halves together.

When you serve the sandwich, it would be fitting to add a tablespoon or two of a rice or lentil salad alongside—something with a fresh taste of grain and perhaps the bite of raisins, nuts, or fine-chopped vegetables mixed into it.

Variations: Sometimes we will add a tablespoon of Greek yogurt to the lemon side, and some extra chopped parsley or cilantro, making a kind of spread. It gives a wonderful freshness—and a little messiness—to the sandwich. If you had some leftover green sauce, or salsa or tartar sauce, they would each be a fine partner on their own to the chicken and avocado.

At the shop:

2 breaded chicken breasts, with their sauce (see page 96)

I loaf French bread, cut into six-inch lengths, or 2 to 4 ciabatta rolls

I lemon

2 to 4 tablespoons chutney, any variety, or plum paste

I ripe avocado

2 tablespoons chopped parsley or cilantro

¼ pound arugula leaves

Salt

Freshly ground pepper

Roasted Beef Tenderloin Ends

SERVES FOUR.

The tenderloin itself is not very flavorful, having little fat and having done little physical work; it is the shock absorber, or bumper guard, at both sides of the animal's back. Italians often serve it when their children are feeling sick, for it is easy to chew and to digest. But it loves to be fussed with. Once you get it dressed up and cooked just to a pink on the inside and blackened outside, it makes a handsome addition, sliced thick, alongside a salad or layered into a sandwich.

You can make this dish with any part of the tenderloin, but the center cut can be expensive. Keep an eye out for the beef ends, the leftover piece where the tenderloin comes to a narrow point. The ends, when not folded and tied back onto the tenderloin, are often sold separately and at considerably less expense than the center cut. Some butchers even blend them into their ground beef. If you can find them, get some, or ask your butcher to hold them for you.

The beef ends cook and absorb flavors best at room temperature, so remove them from the refrigerator 15 minutes before preparing this dish.

At home: Preheat the oven to 400°F.

In a stainless-steel bowl, combine the oil, red-pepper flakes, garlic, paprika or porcini powder, sugar, and salt and black pepper, to taste, and mix together into a paste. Roll the beef in the paste to coat. Add more black pepper. Cover the bowl with a plate or plastic wrap and set aside.

Heat a large ovenproof sauté pan over medium heat for a minute or two. Add a little oil to coat the pan, then add the butter and let it melt until foamy. Do not let the butter brown or burn.

As the butter melts, wipe the excess marinade from the beef ends and lay them, a few at a time, in the pan. They should sizzle and begin to brown but not blacken. Be careful not to overcrowd the pan, or the temperature will drop and the beef will not sear properly. After the beef ends are browned, in 1 to 2 minutes, turn them and brown the other side, 1 to 2 minutes more.

Transfer the pan to the oven. Roast the beef tips for a total of 8 minutes, flipping them halfway through the cooking time. To test for doneness, push on them with your finger for a moment. When they have firmed up, when they do not give in as you push, they should be slightly pink and cooked to medium.

At home:

2 tablespoons olive oil, plus more as needed

Pinch of red-pepper flakes

1 garlic clove, finely chopped

1 teaspoon paprika or porcini mushroom powder

1 tablespoon sugar

Salt

Freshly ground black pepper

1 pound beef tenderloin ends

2 tablespoons butter

½ cup red or white wine

¼ cup warm chicken or beef stock

1 tablespoon tomato paste

½ cup fresh flat-leaf parsley leaves, chopped, plus more as needed

Remove the pan from the oven and set aside on the stove top to rest for 5 minutes. Wrap the hot pan handle in a dishtowel or potholder to protect your hands and the hands of anyone coming in to see what is cooking.

Remove the beef ends from the pan and set them on a warm plate. Pour off the fat in the pan and then add the wine. Set the pan over low heat and cook, scraping the browned bits off the bottom of the pan. As the wine reduces and thickens, add the stock, tomato paste, parsley, and salt and pepper, to taste. Let the sauce bubble and thicken.

Return the ends and any juices that have collected on the plate to the pan and roll them around in the sauce. Add the parsley and some additional pepper, and you are done.

If you are serving them immediately, cut the ends into ½-inch-thick slices across the grain and place 3 or 4 slices on each plate. Pour the sauce over them and sprinkle them with a little extra parsley. Tenderloin loves to luxuriate. If you are taking the ends to work for lunch, pack them, unsliced, in their sauce in an airtight container and refrigerate.

At the shop: Let the ends warm to room temperature and slice them into ½-inch medallions. They can be served with a salad, topped with a lemon vinaigrette, or put into a sandwich (see opposite).

Variations: There are many variations to cooking the tenderloins, for the cut loves the attention. You might chop rosemary and garlic into a paste with olive oil and salt and pepper, and smear that all over the ends before browning them. Or simply wrap them in prosciutto without any seasoning and add slivers of garlic to the pan. Then season them with salt and pepper after cooking.

———————

Roasted Tenderloin Sandwich, Extra-Fancy

SERVES TWO TO FOUR.

We do not have these very often—the beef ends are usually easiest to find during the holidays, when the demand for the center cut is high and the tails are extra. It is a sandwich of good fortune.

At home: Heat a medium saucepan over low heat for a minute, then add the oil, butter, and onions. Stir well, add a good pinch of salt, and cover the pan. Sweat the onions for 20 minutes, stirring once. Uncover the pan, add the sugar, and stir. Cook, stirring frequently, for 25 minutes more. The onions will begin to stick a little and to brown. Add the vinegar, stir, and turn off the heat. Transfer the onions to a storage container, let cool, cover, and refrigerate.

At the shop: Let the tenderloins and browned onions warm up to room temperature.

In a small bowl, mix the horseradish and mayonnaise together, and then stir in the mustard. Add a squirt of lemon juice, stir, and set aside.

Slice the tomato into 8 slices and lightly salt the slices.

Slice the rolls and spread some of the horseradish mayonnaise on one cut side of each. If you have any sauce from the roasted tenderloins, mix that with the butter, and spread the mixture on the other cut side of each roll; otherwise, simply butter the side.

Lay several tenderloin pieces over the horseradish mayonnaise on each roll, slightly overlapping them. Add a little salt and a good grind of pepper. Add 1 Bibb leaf, 2 tomato slices, and a good forkful of the browned onions to each sandwich. Squeeze a little lemon over the onions and close the rolls. Cut each sandwich in half so the layers can be seen, and serve with something fresh, such as peeled carrots or a radish.

At home:

1 tablespoon olive oil

1 tablespoon unsalted butter

1 Walla Walla onion, thinly sliced

Salt

1 tablespoon brown sugar

1 teaspoon balsamic vinegar

At the shop:

1 pound Roasted Beef Tenderloin Ends with their sauce (see page 99), sliced

1 tablespoon horseradish

1 tablespoon mayonnaise

1 teaspoon Colman's dried mustard

½ lemon

1 ripe tomato

Salt

4 ciabatta rolls

1 tablespoon butter, softened

Freshly ground black pepper

1 small head Bibb lettuce, leaves cleaned and dried

Sausages and Ribs, Together Again, with Tomatoes and Sage

SERVES FOUR.

This is a perfect Lunch at the Shop *recipe: It can be easily prepared at home, it can be used at lunch in several ways, and it is a great treat. Typically we use hot Italian sausages, but you should experiment with others, like merguez, boudin, or bratwurst. It is also a treat if you are serving a thick soup, such as a cranberry bean or a lentil (see pages 60 and 74), to stick a rib and a cut of sausage into a corner of the soup.*

At home: Cut the ribs into pairs and pat them dry with a paper towel. Heat a high-sided sauté pan over medium-high heat for 2 minutes. Add the oil and heat for 1 minute. Add the ribs to the pan, skin-side down. They should sizzle. You want to brown them well, so cook them for 3 minutes before turning them. Turn the ribs, then let them cook and brown for 6 to 8 minutes more.

Add the sausages and onions to the pan and stir. Prick the sausages with the tip of a knife. After 2 minutes, add the carrots and celery, stir, and cook, covered, for 10 minutes more, until the sausage has browned. Stir well if any part of the mixture starts to burn.

Place the tomatoes (with juice) in a stainless-steel bowl and break up the tomatoes with your hands, a potato masher, or a large fork. Pour them and their juices into the pan with the ribs, add the sage and garlic, and stir it all very well. Season with salt and pepper, reduce the heat to low, stir again, and cover. Cook, covered, for 45 minutes, but check the pan every 10 minutes, making certain that the mixture is bubbling and not drying out or burning in any spots.

The ribs are done when the meat easily comes off the bone. Taste and add salt and pepper as needed. Add the parsley and the Parmesan.

If not serving immediately, let the dish cool, then transfer to an airtight container and refrigerate.

At the shop: Reheat the dish for 3 minutes in a microwave, or 5 minutes on the stove top over medium heat. Serve with a bowl of rice and a grilled piece of bread. Add plenty of Parmesan and pepper when serving.

At home:

2 to 3 pounds baby back ribs

¼ cup olive oil

1 pound hot or medium fresh Italian sausages, in their casings

1 onion, roughly chopped

1 carrot, roughly chopped

1 celery stalk, roughly chopped

1 can (28 ounces) peeled San Marzano tomatoes (with juice)

1 teaspoon fresh sage, chopped

2 cloves garlic, roughly chopped

Salt

Freshly ground black pepper

½ cup fresh flat-leaf parsley leaves, chopped

2 tablespoons freshly grated Parmesan cheese

At the shop:

1 cup cooked rice

4 slices bread

Freshly grated Parmesan cheese

Freshly ground black pepper

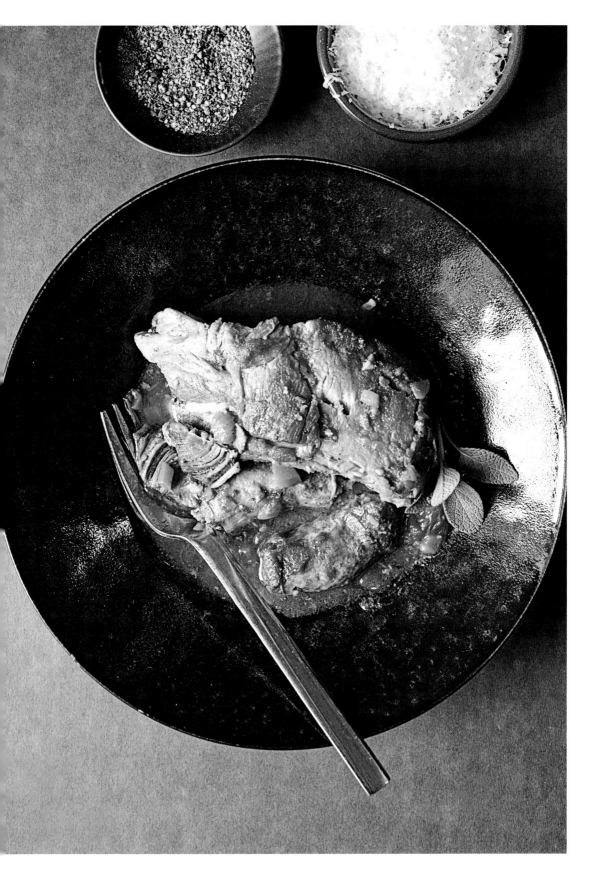

Fish for Tomorrow

SERVES FOUR.

This will take you only a few minutes at home, but it is wonderful at lunch the next day— and a fine recruitment for any tomatoes you need to use.

At home: Pat the fish dry with a paper towel and cut it into 4 equal-size pieces. Place the flour in a shallow bowl or on a plate. Salt and pepper each piece of fish and then dredge it in the flour, shaking off any excess.

Heat a 10-inch sauté pan over medium heat for a moment, then add half of the oil to the pan and heat it for about 2 minutes. You want the oil hot, not scorching. Put half of the fish fillets into the pan (if there is no sizzle when the fish touches the pan, the pan is not hot enough) and cook for 2 minutes to brown one side. Turn the fish over and cook the other side for 2 minutes more. Using a spatula, carefully transfer the cooked fish to a warm plate. Repeat with the remaining pieces of fish, using a touch more oil.

In the same sauté pan, heat the remaining oil. Add the garlic and red-pepper flakes and cook for 2 minutes, being careful not to brown the garlic. Peel and quarter the tomatoes, reserving any juice, and add them to the pan—it should sizzle and bubble a bit. Cook for 1 minute, scraping the pan as it bubbles, then lay all the cooked fish pieces back in the pan. It will be a little crowded. Reduce the heat to low.

If the fillets are thick, they may need 6 to 8 minutes to cook through; if thin, they may only need 4 to 6 minutes. As they say about cooking fish, don't leave early and don't stay late. When the flesh is firm and white, the fish is done.

If you are cooking this for the next day, transfer the fish to a glass container, pour the sauce over the top, add the parsley and thyme, and let cool for 10 minutes before covering and refrigerating.

At the shop: Let the fish come to room temperature for 10 minutes before serving, and crack some black pepper over each piece after plating. Serve the fish with a very green salad.

At home:

1 ½ pounds cod or halibut fillets, skin removed

¼ cup all-purpose flour

Salt

Freshly ground black pepper

¼ cup olive oil

2 garlic cloves, minced

Pinch of red-pepper flakes

4 to 6 ripe tomatoes, or 6 canned tomatoes (with juice)

½ cup fresh flat-leaf parsley leaves, chopped

1 sprig fresh thyme

At the shop:

Freshly ground black pepper

Arugula

½ cup A Very Good Basic Vinaigrette (see page 51)

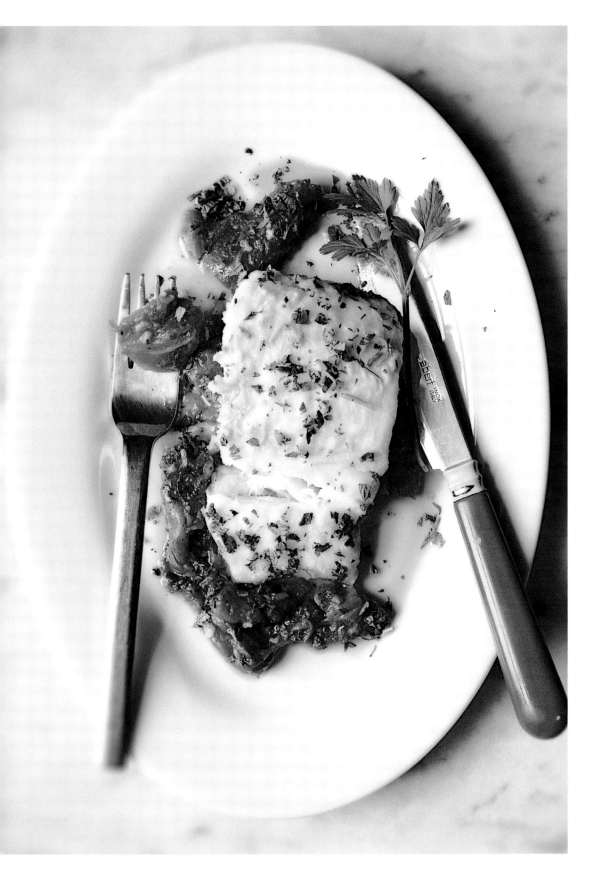

CHAPTER 4

LUNCH IN CONTEXT:
EATING SEASONALLY

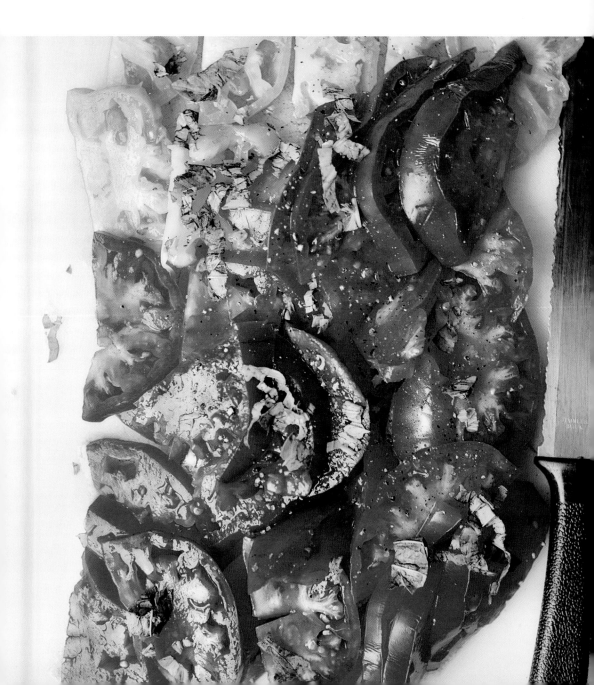

It is not possible to make lunch without keeping the seasons in mind, from the easy bounty of August to the stricter limits of January. You will simply lose track or interest, or both. It is the seasons that set the tone, or the standard, or the possibilities. I asked my friend Markku about the food in Finland. He laughed, remembering that when something came into season, such as blueberries or chanterelles, they would eat that food until it went out of season. His wife, who is from Washington State, said you could get a little tired of the same food and be quietly pleased it was leaving.

While you don't need to take it to extremes, let the season push you a little and give you some direction. Lean on it, use it, take it into account as you plan. Here are some details that might help.

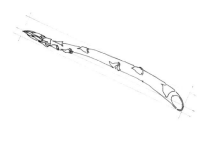

SPRING

As the days warm and lengthen, your options lengthen, as well. The lettuce is much better, the arugula is tender and sweet, and the spinach is at its very best. The chives are finally upright and green-stemmed. Bring all of it into lunch, in sandwiches or floating atop soups and salads.

Your lunches can have less heft, more color, and more specific tastes. As Claudio at our local food shop, DeLaurenti, would often remind me, there is always fresh goat cheese, but it is never as wonderful as in the spring. If you can find some freshly made spring goat cheese, pour good olive oil across it, sprinkle it with fresh chives and rough salt, and know that half the lunch is ready.

Tulips are everywhere but only until June, when they leave for nine months. Buy them for the table—it is a shallow lot who underestimate the gift of flowers.

In spring, pay special attention to:

☐ arugula   ☐ goat cheese   ☐ spring onions

☐ asparagus   ☐ lettuces   ☐ tulips

☐ chives   ☐ peas

☐ fava beans   ☐ spinach

Lentils, Chives, and Goat Cheese: A Handsome Outfit

At the shop:

1 cup Puy lentils, cooked (see page 67)

2 tablespoons fresh chives, finely chopped

6 fresh basil leaves, torn into small pieces

8 arugula leaves, roughly chopped

1 teaspoon fresh lemon juice

Salt

2 tablespoons Greek yogurt

2 tablespoons creamy, fresh goat cheese, at room temperature

Olive oil

Freshly ground black pepper

4 thin slices baguette or dense rye bread

SERVES FOUR.

This dish is the slightest of detail, a toss more than a recipe, a nod to spring.

At the shop: Bring the lentils to room temperature. In a stainless-steel bowl, add half of the chives, the basil, and the arugula to the lentils and toss lightly to combine. Add the lemon juice and toss again. Taste for salt and add as needed.

Mix the yogurt and goat cheese together in a small bowl and fold into the lentils, with only 2 or 3 turns of a fork and spoon. You want the goat cheese and yogurt barely mixed with the rest.

Divide the salad evenly among your 4 largest plates (for this salad, you want some blank space on the plate). Pour a line of oil over each and even a little on the plate itself. Sprinkle the remaining chives and some pepper over each plate, and add a little pinch of salt just off to the side. Be careful that some of the chives and the pepper are spilled off the salad. Serve with very fresh slices of a baguette or thin slices of a dense rye.

THE BRIEF AND BLOODY STRAWBERRIES OF WASHINGTON STATE

They come at the very end of spring, the local strawberries, butting in between days of sun and days of wind and rain, and if the sun has the upper hand, they will be ready by the middle of June. The Washington local strawberry is a very dark red, breasted from the rain of a too-long wet spring. All ten of your fingers will be stained red if you eat them out of hand.

There are other strawberries all around them. The California strawberries have been out for two months and are designed to go for another two months, and there is an ever-bearing variety in Washington that will have berries until October.

But this local berry, it is a different sort—it will only be here for two weeks and then is gone until next spring. They are too fragile to march deeper into the summer, but they are the best strawberries of them all. A pure strawberry taste, a soft flesh—simply mashed slightly together, they are a strawberry sauce.

They travel poorly, so they are never exported; they are only local. You can hold them a bit in the freezer, or by saucing them with sugar, or by making jam, and they are happy allies for all of that. But the greatest privilege is to eat them while they are fresh.

It is a good habit for a town to know when its fruits and vegetables are best—especially during a time when our culture is so rapidly paving over its seasons.

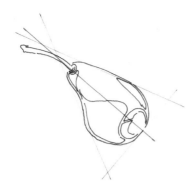

SUMMER

In the summer, you have the task of deciding what to combine, what to celebrate. There are always lettuces to buy during the rest of the year, but none have flourished in your local sunshine. Give your lunches the luxury of summer: the fresh greens, of course, but also the true young carrots, the early beets, the fresh basil, and the real tomatoes.

Keep the salad dressings simple, taking care that the oil, vinegar, peppercorns, and salt are all fresh and first-rate. Prepare a summer salad with the greens first. Set the greens on their plates, then add any feta or bits of chicken or fish to the bowl you mixed your dressing in and lay them on top, to keep the different parts more on their own. Use the colors as they come: the strawberries to the raspberries to the blackberries, the bright peas to the broccoli to the green beans. And for a couple of months, for their high season, keep basil and mint on hand, buying them fresh every three or four days and tossing them into soups and pastas and salads. Chop them, singly or together, with or without salt, and mix in olive oil to pour over fish and fresh cheese or tomatoes and onions.

In the summer, don't forget to stock up on:

☐ basil   ☐ dahlias   ☐ potatoes

☐ blueberries   ☐ garlic   ☐ raspberries

☐ broccoli   ☐ green beans   ☐ strawberries

☐ chanterelles   ☐ greens/lettuces   ☐ tomatoes

☐ cherries   ☐ mint

☐ corn   ☐ peaches

Chanterelles, Onions, Potatoes, and Eggs

At home:

2 pounds Yukon Gold, Yellow Finn, or similar potatoes

Salt

½ cup olive oil

2 yellow onions, halved and thinly sliced

2 eggs

Freshly ground black pepper

½ cup fresh flat-leaf parsley leaves, chopped

2 tablespoons butter

1 pound chanterelles, cleaned, brushed, and quartered

10 to 12 cherry tomatoes

½ teaspoon garlic, finely chopped

¼ cup freshly grated Parmesan cheese

At the shop:

2 cups arugula

½ cup A Very Good Basic Vinaigrette (see page 51)

Salt

Freshly ground black pepper

¼ cup freshly grated Parmesan cheese

SERVES FOUR.

This will seem like a lot of work, but it is more detail than actual labor. The difficulty is that you must find good chanterelles. Good ones are like a lovely pile of fresh daffodils, and bad ones are like a pile of wet bathing-suit bottoms. Should only the wet-bathing-suit variety be available, lay them carefully out on a wire rack. Turn them every couple of hours until they dry and regain their form.

Chanterelles are a gift. They grow in summer and fall, amid fir and pine and in coastal climates, only in places with four seasons. They are beloved—and mourned—in Europe, for pollution has cut deeply into their habitat. In Germany in the fall, the vegetable markets now all display Washington State chanterelles. The tradition for pfifferlingen (chanterelles in German) stretches back many generations in German cooking. In Washington State, the tradition of chanterelles has only just begun—we are still learning the great fortune of our mushroom bounty. Washington mushrooms are already enjoyed around the world, but some American cooks are still hesitant to put them to use.

The French food industry has spent a fortune trying to cultivate chanterelles and bring them into a controllable supply, yet all efforts have failed completely. The mushroom simply grows of its own accord, returning each year. Some years, the chanterelle is as common as a potato, and others, it is as rare as a true king salmon.

If it is summer or fall, and you can find chanterelles, this is a good recipe for enjoying them—and a wonderful meal the next day at lunch.

Chanterelles, like all mushrooms, are like a sponge to moisture. You never wash them; you only wipe them off with a cloth to clean them. The early chanterelle is likely drier than the one a month later. When you are sautéing them, you must keep in mind just how much moisture they have; it will affect how to cook them. If they release a lot of liquid as they are heated, then you must stay with them, even turning the heat up a little. If you go too slowly, they will simply cook into a limp mass. If they do not release any liquid, then you may even need to add a couple of tablespoons of chicken stock or pasta-cooking water.

At home: Place the potatoes and a little salt in a saucepan and add cool water to cover them by 1 inch. Bring the water to a boil over medium-high heat, then turn the heat down a bit and cook the potatoes for 15 minutes. Drain the potatoes and set aside.

Heat a 12-inch sauté pan over low heat for a moment and then add ¼ cup of the oil and three-quarters of the onions. Cover and cook, stirring occasionally, for 20 minutes, or until the onions are translucent. Do not brown them.

Crack the eggs into a small bowl, beat them lightly, season with salt and pepper, and set aside. Slice the cooked potatoes and add them to the pan with the onions. Shake the pan well, season with salt and pepper, and increase the heat to medium. Cook, uncovered, for 6 to 8 minutes, until the potatoes and onions have browned. Remove the pan from the heat, quickly stir in the eggs, and then return the pan to the heat. Cook, stirring, for about 1 minute, until the eggs have cooked and begin to brown. Remove the pan from the heat, add half of the parsley and 2 grinds of pepper, and let stand for 1 to 2 minutes. Transfer the mixture to a warmed flat oval or round serving dish.

Clean and dry the pan, if necessary, and set it back over medium heat. Add the remaining ¼ cup oil, 1 tablespoon of the butter, and the remaining onions. Stir well and cook for 3 minutes, then add the chanterelles, season with salt and pepper, and stir to coat the mushrooms in the oil and onion. It will seem like a large pile of mushrooms, but they do cook down a little. Keep them moving so they cook evenly.

Sauté the mushrooms, tossing and stirring as you go, for about 6 minutes. You will smell a slight mocha scent when they are nearly done, and they should have begun to slightly stick to the pan. Toss in the cherry tomatoes, add a tablespoon of water, and reduce the heat to low. Remove the pan from the heat and spoon the mushrooms and tomatoes over the potatoes on the serving platter.

Return the pan to the heat and add the remaining 1 tablespoon butter, some of the remaining parsley, and the garlic to the pan. Quickly stir to bring it all together (if it is too dry at this point, add a little warmed water). Pour the sauce over the mushrooms. Add the remaining parsley and the Parmesan.

If you are serving the mushrooms the next day, let everything cool, then cover the platter well with plastic wrap (you do not want errant refrigerator smells joining the spongelike mushrooms) and refrigerate overnight.

At the shop: Bring the platter of potatoes and mushrooms to room temperature. Mix the arugula with the vinaigrette in a large stainless-steel bowl. Taste and season with salt and pepper—especially pepper—as needed, then add the Parmesan to the salad. Do this quickly and lightly, and then, with tongs, lay the arugula over the mushrooms and potatoes.

Variation: You could make this dish with cultivated white button mushrooms available at every grocer. Do considerably less tossing and stirring as you sauté. You want the buttons to brown a bit. And because the buttons are cultivated, they will not release much liquid. When you go back to make the sauce, add ½ cup hot chicken or vegetable stock to the pan and add a sprig of thyme to the sauce. The buttons do not have the subtlety of the chanterelles; they know only the basement, not the woods.

KNOWING ONE APPLE FROM ANOTHER

I learned a lot about apples one day at the doctor's office. In the waiting room, on a lovely and impatient fall day, I began talking to a woman from south Seattle about making apple pie. The weather had been perfect for months—a hot August, a few late summer rainfalls, then cold nights and warm September days. The market was filled with apples.

I asked what her favorite apples for pie were. She laughed and told me what it was like to be an eighteen-year-old girl fifty years ago.

"We all knew probably sixteen different apples—we knew them by smell and sight and taste. You had to. You knew the ones that came in late August: They were fine for sauce and cider, but only a fool would use them for pies. They could not hold up. We knew the Liberties were not due until October, but you could always taste a pie that had Liberty apples in them.

"The Gravensteins were everywhere, but you had to mix them with winesaps to get the right taste and some Romes to keep the texture, or all you had was mush under that crust.

"Now, of course, none of my kids knows one apple from another, and they expect them to be the same every month. But even so, when I can find some Sierra Beauties, and lay them out on the table, they will be gone in a day. My kids still have good taste."

In 1905, there were more than two hundred varieties of apples grown in Washington State. By 1982, there were only two varieties in abundance, Golden and Red Delicious. But now, Washington State lists more than one hundred varieties available commercially. It is getting better.

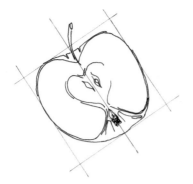

FALL

———

By fall, with luck, the weather will hold, and the tomatoes will sweeten even further. The cool nights will mean that arugula and spinach that wilted in the summer heat can return, for a moment. If you see them at the farmers' market, get them. Soon the greens will all be coming from greenhouses. Sunflowers are the color of fall, as are the squashes and pumpkins. And with beans, by fall, you can slowly give more heft to your soups, adding chard and the potatoes that are just coming up. The basil is gone, but a spoonful of pesto on a bean soup or a broth will recollect the summer.

It is the time of zucchini and eggplant, the longer-growing sorts. You can work them into a lunch, but some of the preparation will first need to be done at home— grilling or roasting or frying—for these are end-of-season vegetables, a bit heartier, not delicate enough to be eaten raw. Keep them well-covered when refrigerated (or they will take on smells from the fridge), and bring them to room temperature before serving. They are glad for any attention—mint or garlic, parsley or thyme, or yogurt.

If you can find good apples and pears, bring them into lunch. Sliced, with soft or hard cheeses, with dabs of fig paste; cut up, with raisins and fresh walnuts and feta; as applesauce, from the earliest or sourest apples, sweetened with sugar. There are always apples, but fresh apples are only here for a month or two. Find a bottle of maple syrup, true maple syrup, and pour only a very little of it over pear and apple slices, or on applesauce that is over the pear and apple slices.

In fall, set your table with:

- [ ] apples
- [ ] asters
- [ ] brussels sprouts
- [ ] eggplant

- [ ] grapes
- [ ] late tomatoes
- [ ] maple syrup
- [ ] pears

- [ ] pumpkin
- [ ] squash
- [ ] sunflowers

White Bean Soup and Broccoli Rabe

SERVES FOUR.

This is a wonderful and very easy dish to make. But it is like commuting: You must plan a bit for the best way to get there. This dish is very good the next day, but you must keep it refrigerated and well-covered. And you must heat it deliberately. It is not meant to sit over low heat for more than a minute or two.

The fresh beans are all gone by the fall, but the farmers' markets often have dried beans that are wonderful for this dish. The broccoli rabe gives the soup a heartiness suited for cooler days.

At home: In a medium saucepan, heat 2 tablespoons of the oil over medium-low heat. Add the garlic and cook until softened, about 4 minutes—do not brown the garlic. Add the beans—they should sizzle just a bit. Stir them well to coat them in the oil, and season with salt and pepper. Cover the pan and reduce the heat to low. Cook for 5 minutes.

With a slotted spoon, remove one-third of the beans and process them through a ricer back into the saucepan. Add half of the stock and stir until the mash thickens the stock.

Rinse the broccoli rabe and shake or spin it dry. Chop it into 1-inch pieces—stalk, floret, and leaves—and toss them into the saucepan with the beans. Add a good pinch of salt and stir. The heat from the beans will cook the broccoli rabe. Be certain to stir often. If the mixture gets too thick, add a bit more warm stock. Taste after 6 minutes; the beans should be a little creamy, the broccoli rabe should not be mushy. Taste for salt and season, as needed; you do not want this dish to be bland. Let the dish cool, and then transfer it to an airtight container and refrigerate it.

At the shop: Loosen the mixture with heated water before putting it in the microwave. Serve the warm beans and broccoli rabe with a drizzle of oil across the top, the parsley, and the Parmesan.

At home:

2 tablespoons olive oil

2 garlic cloves, finely chopped

1 cup dried white beans (cannellini or petite French beans), cooked and drained (see page 59)

Salt

Freshly ground black pepper

1 cup warm chicken or vegetable stock

½ pound broccoli rabe

At the shop:

2 tablespoons olive oil

2 tablespoons fresh flat-leaf parsley leaves, chopped

½ cup freshly grated Parmesan cheese

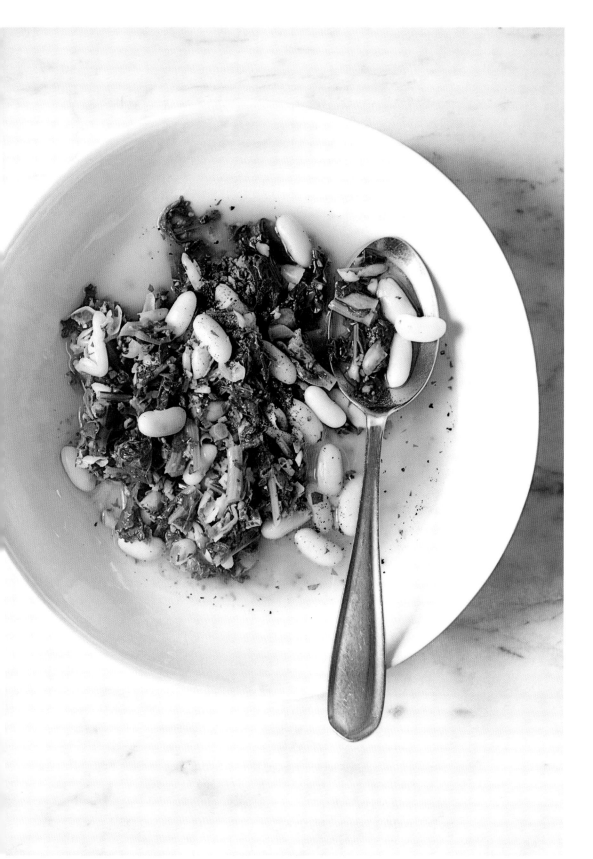

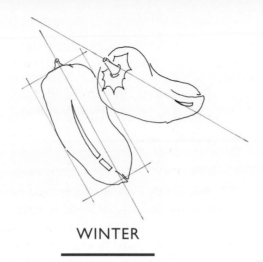

WINTER

In winter, make a particular note to buy fresh parsley and lemons. They are easy enough to find year-round, and they lighten the sense of a meal and whistle the strains of other, lighter seasons. *Prezzemolo*, "parsley" in Italian, chopped quite fine and sauced with good olive oil and some salt, will help make any soup fresher and lovelier. The lemon helps if for no other reason than its color. I am always pleased to see it on the counter; it means there are many things I can do. A few drops of lemon juice will revive a piece of fish, a slice of chicken, even a meatball. You can mince a thin lemon peel with parsley and salt and sprinkle it over pasta or lentils. It is a taste that trims the weight of a food and a color that only sunlight can raise—and those are fine allies in winter.

For cold climates, the winter meals will dig deeper into stews, beans, meats, and pastas. January can be a long haul, hard on both food and one's spirits, so bring some help. Roasted red peppers, marinated in a little garlic and hot pepper, take only scant preparation. Carrots are used to the cold—peel them, or cook them with sugar, salt, and butter at home, and eat them cold at the shop.

And seafood, too, knows cold. Much of the freshest and brightest winter product is seafood. Where it may be fragile and mushy in the warm seasons, crabs and clams, sole and cod are at their best in the cold, hampered only by the task of harvesting them.

In winter, these can be a great help:

☐ beets	☐ clams	☐ roasted red peppers
☐ carrots	☐ flat-leaf parsley	☐ roses (in January; they get more expensive in February)
☐ cauliflower	☐ lemons and limes	
☐ cilantro	☐ lentils	☐ soups

Pasta with Fresh Clams
(*Spaghetti alle Vongole*)

This is very easy to make well if you have good clams, good garlic, fresh parsley, fresh bread crumbs, and very good spaghetti. Everything is out in the open with this dish.

We make this quite often. I am always surprised at how good it is the next day, and I am not its only supporter. When I make this dish to bring in for lunch, I must also make enough to leave two servings at home. The clams, the broth, and even the bread crumbs seem perfectly happy to be reheated. The winter clams are considerably hardier, and their juice is clear.

Any time you serve a seafood pasta, keep in mind that a salad afterward can help to balance the tastes. It need not be an elaborate production, but the greens, and the acidity of vinegar or lemon, can be particularly welcome.

At home: Bring a large pot of salted water to a boil.

Add the pasta to the boiling water. It should take about 10 minutes to cook, and you want it a minute or so underdone so you can continue to cook it with the clams. You must be nimble for this dish.

Heat a wide saucepan or paella pan over medium heat for 30 seconds. Add ¼ cup of the oil, the garlic, and the red-pepper flakes and cook for just 30 seconds (do not burn the garlic), then add the clams and stir well. Cook for 1 minute, then add the white wine (it should sizzle), shake the pan well, and cover the pan; you are off to the races.

Stir the spaghetti; it should be only half done. Check on the clams; if they are fresh, they may take only 3 minutes to open. Uncover the pan and remove any open clams with tongs; set them aside in a bowl. Things get busy at this point. The rest of the clams are all about to open, the pasta is nearly done, and you still need to scrape the clams out of their shells. Do it quickly, or have someone help you. Set the clam meat aside in a bowl.

If you have everything in order, or are lucky, then all the clams have been removed (any that do not open are dead—throw them away). Drain the pasta and very quickly add it to the still-cooking clam sauce.

The starchy pasta will thicken the clam sauce in only a minute or so, and the instant that starts to happen, add the meat from the clams

At home:

Salt

½ pound spaghetti

½ cup olive oil

2 cloves garlic, minced or finely chopped

½ teaspoon red-pepper flakes

2 pounds small manila clams, scrubbed with cold water and kept cold in a colander

½ cup dry white wine

½ cup fresh flat-leaf parsley leaves, finely chopped

Freshly ground black pepper

1 cup fresh toasted bread crumbs (see page 143)

At the shop:

Olive oil

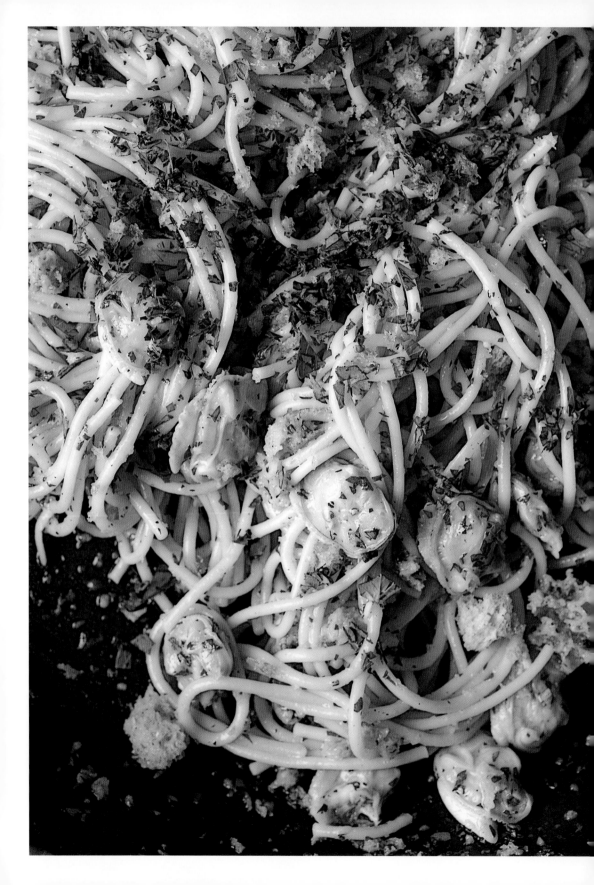

and the parsley. Toss or stir or fold it all together, taste and add salt and pepper, then add the bread crumbs. Remove the pan from the heat and add a ⅛ cup of oil. The *vongole* is ready to serve.

If it is being prepared for serving the next day, let it cool, then transfer it to a deep glass container with a tight lid. Scrape any of the leftover parsley or bread crumbs over the top, cover the dish, and refrigerate it.

At the shop: You will need to microwave the dish, but be careful to get the serving bowls warm, as well. Just before serving, add a drizzle of oil.

———————

CHAPTER 5

TIMES OF INVENTION:
MAKING LUNCH WITH THE NEIGHBORHOOD

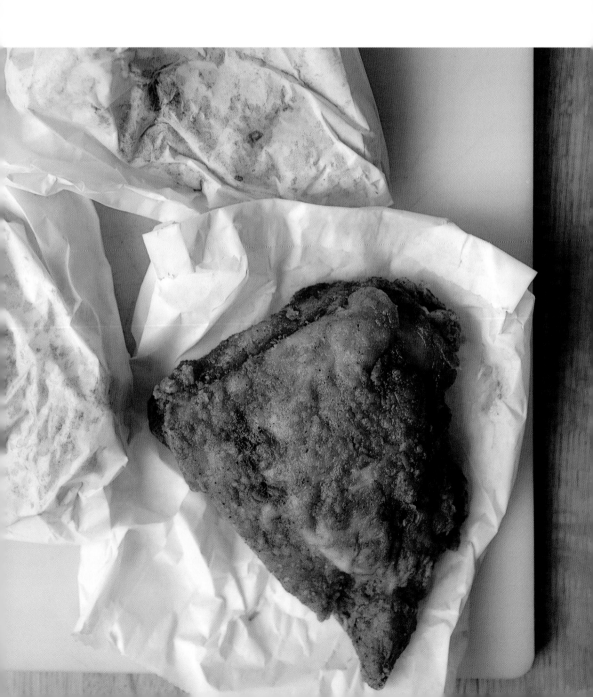

There will be times when, for whatever reason, you have nothing prepared or saved for lunch. But you still have lunch to serve. You may need to pick up a few items—an avocado, some lettuce, or a few rolls—but the dishes in this chapter are quick and easy to assemble, and everything can be done at the shop.

At such times when we have nothing planned for lunch, we improvise and go foraging. You could, of course, simply buy lunch and bring it back. But you have the simple equipment and ingredients to explore a little and make new combinations—whatever you put together will surely be more varied, and more personal, than its parts. In a way, you are eating in the neighborhood.

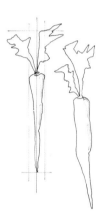

TEN ITEMS AND PROBABLY FEWER

When we are in a mood, good or bad, driven outside by too much sun or no sun at all, when the food in the refrigerator has lost too much charm, when it is time for a little air, we head out to the neighborhood or farther afield and make up lunch as we go.

This is, of course, an easy task if the farmers' market has just opened for the season. (I walk through the Union Square Greenmarket in Manhattan to meet my publisher and editor and always think how lucky they are.) But it can also be done with a grocery store or shop by shop.

Whatever the season, there are always possibilities. Start with bread, if you can find some, and since you are on a hunt, let it be the loaf you never try: the one with olives or potato or the Balkan sourdough starter. If there are no breads that lure you, move to pita bread or tortillas. But for those, you must have a sauce or the makings of a sauce: yogurt, parsley, perhaps a lemon, or hummus.

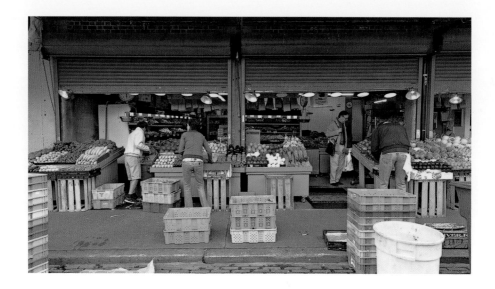

There are always a few avocados. And a lime. Even some celery. Now look for a
hot soup, preferably one that has been creamed or smoothed, for you will use it as a
base. There are chickpea soups, lentil soups, tomato soups, barley soups, and bean
soups that seem to have endured the craze to modernism, and they will all work. We
avoid cheese soups—too sweet.

Once you have the base, then you can poke around for one more item: perhaps
a small container of pasta salad, or some roasted potatoes, barbecued pork, or even a
slice of pepperoni pizza. Our surprise find one day was a fresh seafood ceviche from a
tiny fish market. They made it on Thursdays and Fridays only, as much for their own
lunch as for their customers.

Heat the soup, taste it for salt and pepper, and then consider what to add and
how to add it. The pasta salad can go right into most soups; the heat will take the chill
off. Hold the liquid from the salad back; it is likely too acidic. The potatoes can go on
their own or with a little barbecued pork. And cut the pizza slice into one-inch strips
and sink them into the soup.

Then consider your avocado and the celery. They are both wonderful alongside
a quick lunch, sliced and lightly salted, with a little lime squirted on them. But taste
your soup; that may be just the place for some thin slices of avocado and/or celery.
Finish with fresh pepper. You can mush up a little avocado to make a spread and add
that to whatever bread or pita you found. Squeeze a little lime on that, as well. And if
you should find a ceviche, it is a great surprise how wonderful it tastes in an otherwise
routine cream-of-potato soup.

A MOST FREQUENT GUEST

Our most frequent and yet elusive guest for lunch is Paul Maritz. He loves food, he hates pomp, and a lunch at the shop is his kind of urban secret. He often tells other people about it but never precisely how it works or how it is possible. And so far, no one has come in after him.

He always calls, but only thirty minutes before—enough time for him to stop at the Italian food market, the wine shop, and Frank's Quality Produce, to pick up a few things from the neighborhood. He knows full well we have whatever else is needed.

Paul was one of the early veterans at Microsoft, before there even was a public Internet. At first, we only knew him as Ben's dad. Ben was employed at the shop as a stock boy. We had little stock, but soon he was fiddling with our lone computer.

Having watched us thumb through thousands of file cards for book titles and inventory, Ben wrote a program to run the shop. It had a few typos (*sucsessfully*), and still does, but we also still operate with it. Ben hand-carried us though the Stygian tunnels of the Internet and then went on to college, graduate school, marriage, and fatherhood. And still, when he is back in Seattle, he will make time to sit in the back of the shop and set up for a lunch.

When Ben left for college, Paul, realizing we would soon sink into shallow, murky water, took over the stewardship of the bookstore computer, becoming perhaps the most overqualified IT repairman in history—by then, he was the vice president of Platforms Strategy and one of five members on its executive management team. (He has since assigned the bookstore custodial work to younger tech souls and gone forth to joust in the Cloud.)

Having come first from Zimbabwe and then Microsoft, Paul has a finely honed enmity and distrust of marketing or salesmanship. He would never ask a shop clerk, "Which of the cheeses do you recommend?" Instead, he simply buys a selection: some sliced meats, olives, and pickled onions; then some figs and dates; some cherries when they finally arrive, and oranges; and a couple of bottles of Barolo, a trustworthy and firm Italian red wine.

He knows we often have the best bread in the neighborhood, and we will always have good butter, some chutney, some greens, maybe a pasta or two, mustard, salt, and the humor to feel that guests are an honor.

There are times we must leave him nearly alone, for we have too much to do that day; other times we take his presence as a sign to give that day up. Paul is fine either way—he is there for lunch at the shop.

One Mondo Burrito for the Table

1 big burrito (takeout)

2 tablespoons balsamic vinegar

Salt

½ cup olive oil

Freshly ground black pepper

8 ounces mixed greens

4 ounces feta cheese (optional)

1 ripe avocado, halved, pitted, peeled, and sliced

¼ cup salsa, red or green (purchased, or see page 35)

½ cup cilantro and/or fresh flat-leaf parsley, stems removed

The Mondo burrito, or any extra-large Mexican-style selection, is surely a takeaway from the "big is always better" SUV theme, but it is often too big for one person. We have deconstructed one and been pleased to extend it to four servings.

We have a lovely Mexican grocery shop nearby. They do not make salads or Mondo burritos, but they do make wonderful small tacos to go, with their own rice and beans and salsa. Often we will buy a dozen of their tacos and add them to this salad instead of the burrito.

Cut the burrito into 4 equal pieces with a serrated knife.

In a small bowl, combine 1 tablespoon of vinegar and some salt and let the salt dissolve, then stir the oil into the vinegar with a fork. Keep stirring and add a couple of drops of water—it will help emulsify the dressing. When it is smooth, crack fresh pepper into it. Put the greens into a stainless-steel bowl, pour the dressing over them, and toss quickly and lightly. Divide the greens among 4 dinner plates, placing them lightly in the center of each plate.

Put 1 piece of burrito cut-side up on each plate, to the side of the salad. Crumble the cheese, if using, in the salad bowl and toss it with the dressing left in the bowl. Spoon the cheese over the burrito and greens. Salt the avocado slices and lay them over the salad. Put the salsa where it will look best. Add the remaining balsamic vinegar in drops on the avocado, where it can be seen. Chop and sprinkle the cilantro and/or parsley over it all.

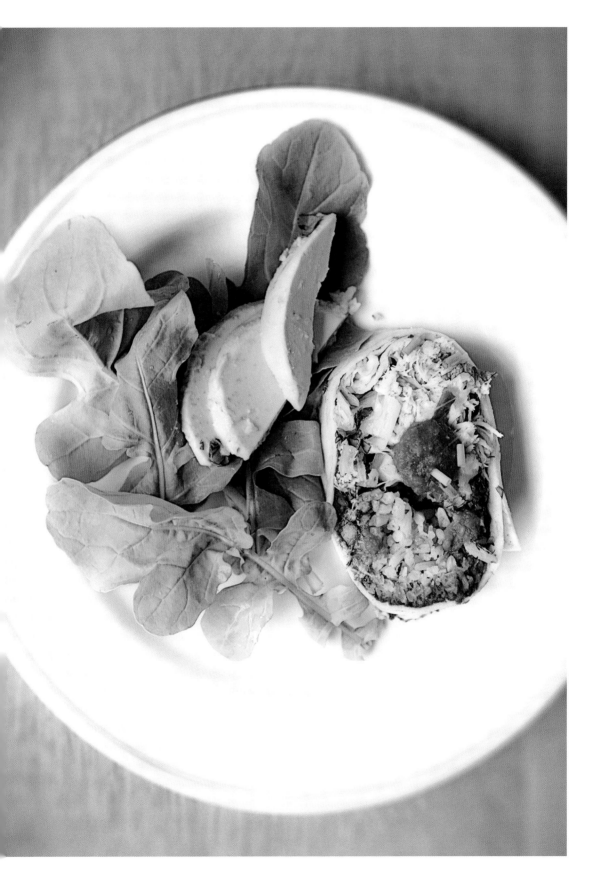

Sushi to Go, with Others for Lunch

SERVES FOUR.

1 lemon

Salt

½ cup olive oil

A few drops of sesame oil

1 head Bibb lettuce

1 nigiri or maki sushi selection, tuna or salmon (takeout)

Soy sauce

Wasabi

Freshly ground black pepper

1 navel or blood orange, cut into wedges

1 ripe avocado, halved, pitted, peeled, and sliced (optional)

Many markets now have sushi available in their to-go cases. Pay close attention to the origin of the sushi package and its date. There are some wonderful small suppliers who sell their sushi to go and take great pride in keeping their offers fresh and well-rotated. In truth, sushi was never meant to sit in a to-go cooler. But if you choose carefully, sushi can involve wonderful ingredients, carefully prepared, and that is what you are adding to your lunch. The to-go containers typically have soy sauce and wasabi, which you will need for this dish, already packed inside them.

Squeeze half of the lemon into a small bowl, add some salt, and let it sit for 2 minutes to dissolve. Add the oil and stir with a fork until it emulsifies. Taste it—the lemon should account for 30 percent of the taste. Stir in a drop or two of sesame oil. If the greens are large, tear them into smaller pieces, and toss them quickly in the dressing. Divide the dressed greens among 4 plates.

Without disrespecting the sushi (in fact, sympathizing with its lonely spot in a plastic case with plastic grass), rearrange the pieces individually on the lettuce, often bisecting them first. Dot the sushi pieces with soy sauce and tiny dabs of wasabi. Add a touch of black pepper. Add avocado to the plate, if using. Arrange the orange wedges on a plate nearby.

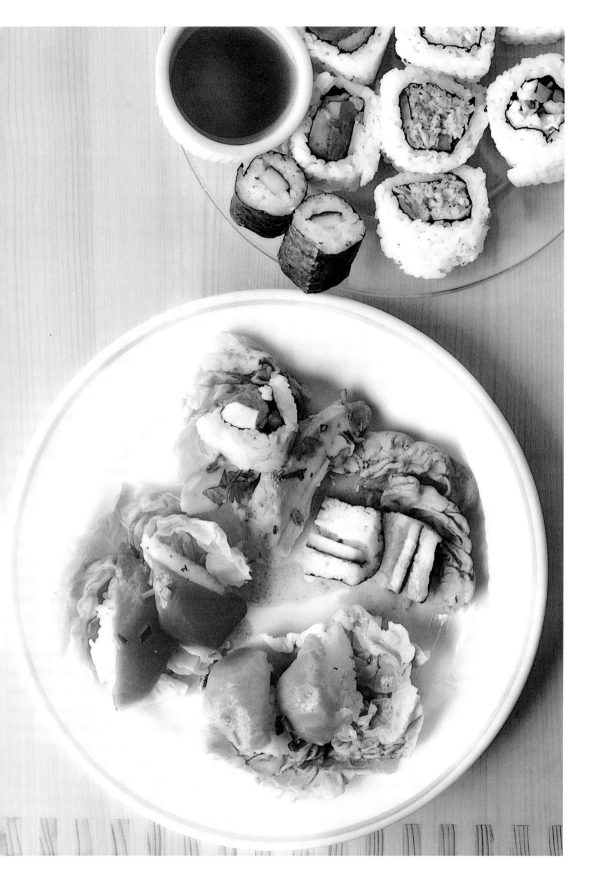

Fried Chicken Sandwich, Your Own Way

SERVES FOUR.

6 deep-fried chicken thighs, or 1 breast piece and 2 thighs

¼ cup olive oil

¼ cup mixed fresh flat-leaf parsley and cilantro, stems removed, chopped

Salt

Freshly ground black pepper

1 ripe avocado, halved and pitted

1 lemon

4 hamburger or hotdog rolls

2 tablespoons mayonnaise

1 ripe tomato, chopped into small pieces and salted

8 ounces arugula

Some days need a guilty addition of crispness.

Deep-frying can disguise almost anything, so try to choose a shop that is actively cooking chicken, not letting it sit around. This is a wonderful sandwich for a Friday, when people's spirits might need a lift. The crispy pieces combined with the tomato, arugula, lemon, and soft bread are wonderful. Serve this sandwich immediately, while the different textures are intact.

When I am making this, I always think that the fried-chicken markets should make it, as well. It is a small but true antidote to deep-frying.

With your fingers, pull the chicken meat and skin from the bones, and put the meat into a bowl. Cut the meat into finger-size strips, removing any leftover bone or gristle.

Mix the oil with half of the parsley and cilantro and stir with a fork. Add salt and pepper and stir some more. Taste it—you need to be able to taste the salt and the oil.

With a tablespoon, scoop out the avocado into a small bowl. Mash it a little, and then add salt and pepper, the juice of half of the lemon, and a pinch of the parsley and cilantro.

Split the rolls and spoon the parsley mixture and the mayonnaise on both inner sides. Lay some of the fried chicken pieces on one side and some of the avocado on top of the chicken. Spoon the tomatoes onto the other roll, and place a handful of arugula over that. Season with salt and pepper and a squeeze of lemon on both sides, and close the rolls. The arugula should stick out in several directions.

Variation: You can create this sandwich just as easily with fried fish, especially cod, and especially with smaller pieces. But be ready to make it before you get the fish, and make it quickly, so the fish will still have its crispiness. Use a bit more lemon and salt when serving fish.

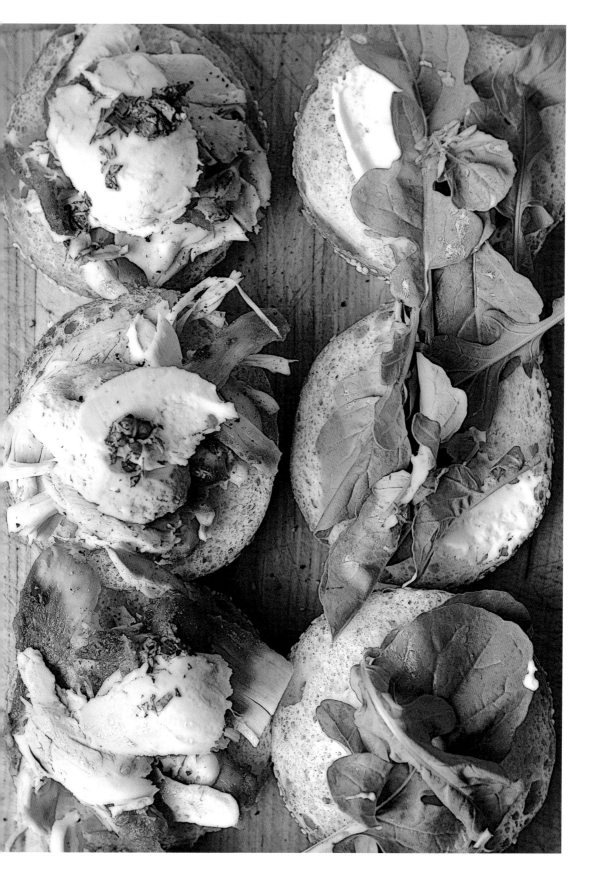

CHAPTER 6

A WEEK OR TWO:
A PLAN FOR THE LUNCHES

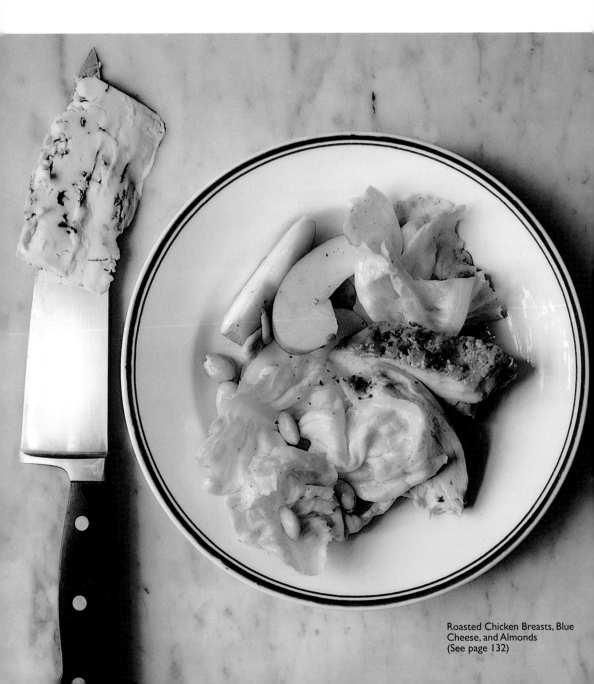

Roasted Chicken Breasts, Blue
Cheese, and Almonds
(See page 132)

What follows is a suggested menu for ten workdays, or two weeks, including variations. As you get into a pattern of making lunch, the separate menus will blur a bit and cross over. You will have a little too much left of this and not enough of that. You will adjust a little; that is the nature of lunch.

There may also be days that a little yogurt and an apple are more than enough—you can catch up to the menu later. But this is a start. You may not need it all, or you can lean on it and know that, for two weeks, lunch is in hand.

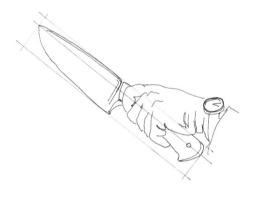

WEEK 1

For the first week, you have a pasta, a lentil soup, some chicken, some sausage, salmon, and a couscous. They all involve some work at home and some constructing at work, but none of them is labor intensive.

At the shop, you will need—as always, really—to keep parsley on hand, and to have a supply of Parmesan, some mayonnaise, a lemon, olive oil, vinegar, and good salt and pepper.

There are a few particulars you will need this week: cornichons, dill, mint, feta cheese, apples, Bibb lettuce, blue cheese, and marcona almonds. Also, Greek yogurt, a ripe avocado, and some pita bread. You may not need all of this at once, but, by the end of the week, whatever you have left can join up with the couscous.

Roasted Chicken Breasts, Blue Cheese, and Almonds

SERVES FOUR.

At the shop:

2 tablespoons A Very Good Basic Vinaigrette (see page 51)

1 small head Bibb lettuce

½ pound Spanish marcona almonds

2 fresh apples, sliced, sprinkled with lemon juice and a bit of sugar

2 skinless, roasted chicken breasts, at room temperature (see page 91)

Salt

Fresh lemon juice

½ pound Oregon blue cheese

There is always a jumble to the start of a week, and this is a lunch where you grab what you have and hope it works. For the Monday meal, use the simplest way to roast a chicken breast, described on page 91—you can cook the two breasts the day before, while doing all the other things that Sunday often calls for.

You can also incorporate any leftovers, such as roasted potatoes or vegetables, from your Sunday dinner. What makes this all work are the ingredients and their freshness. The Bibb is always a reliable host, and almonds and blue cheese are always wonderful guests.

Buy extra blue cheese and apples, and slices of each could go on a plate and be the dessert. Or save them—you have meals coming up, such as the lentil soup or the couscous, that could use the bite of the blue cheese or the crispness of the apple.

At the shop: Place the dressing in a large stainless-steel bowl and add the lettuce. Toss to coat, then lift the greens out of the bowl with tongs, and lay a few on each of 4 plates.

Toss the almonds and half of the apples in the leftover dressing, and place them around the greens on each plate. Do all of this with some haste—you do not want the greens or apples drenched in oil; you want their appearance to signal freshness.

Lay the chicken breast on a cutting board, and cut the breast on a slight diagonal into ¾-inch slices.

Lightly salt and sprinkle a bit of lemon juice onto the chicken, and lay the pieces around the salad (not on top, or it will plop the thing down). Cut off one-quarter of the blue cheese. Put it on a little plate and break it up with a fork, then divide the pieces evenly among the plates.

Penne Pasta with Sausage, Red Peppers, and Peas

SERVES FOUR TO SIX PEOPLE.

Ever since the chef Peter Cipra (see page 134) made this for us, it has been a favorite at the shop. The penne loves this sauce; peas and bits of bell pepper and cream get up into the tube, and the Parmesan melts a bit onto the ridges of the penne. This was meant to be a cold-weather dish. Boil a little extra pasta and reserve 1 cup for Wednesday's lunch.

At home: Bring a large pot of water to a boil. Salt the water once it has come to a boil.

Heat a 12- or 14-inch sauté pan over medium heat for 2 minutes. Add the oil and, 15 seconds later, add the butter. A minute later, after the butter has melted but not browned, add the onions. Toss them to coat in the oil and butter, then add the sausage and peppers, and toss again. Cook, tossing frequently, for 6 to 8 minutes. Watch closely to make sure it does not burn—the sausages should brown but not blacken.

When the sausages are browned and the onion is golden, season with salt and pepper and add the tomatoes. Stir well, then deglaze the pan with ½ cup of the boiling salted water ladled from the pot. Stir to combine, then reduce the heat and let the tomatoes cook.

Add the pasta to the boiling water and cook for 10 to 12 minutes. Penne is a bit heavy and tends to sink at first, so be certain to stir it to break up any clumps.

Stir the sausage mixture, add the peas, and stir again. Add ½ cup of the pasta water to the pan and stir, then add the cream. Keep stirring—you are trying to both incorporate the cream and slightly thicken it, so keep the heat moderate. Cook for a minute or two at the most. Remove the pan from the heat, toss in half the Parmesan, and stir. Taste and add more pepper and salt, if needed.

The pasta should be done. Drain it quickly, reserving some of the cooking water and 1 cup of the pasta for tomorrow's lunch. If your pan is big enough, toss the still-wet pasta into the pan. If you do not have room, then toss the wet pasta into a big, heated pan. Salt the pasta, and add half of the remaining Parmesan while it is still very hot. Mix the sauce into the pasta. If it seems dry, add some of the reserved pasta cooking water, stirring all the time. Add the remaining cheese and the parsley, and that should be it.

At home:

Salt

½ cup olive oil

4 tablespoons butter

1 yellow onion, sliced very thin

4 hot or sweet Italian sausages, cut crosswise into 1-inch pieces

1 red bell pepper, stemmed, seeded, and cut into ¼-inch slices

1 yellow bell pepper, stemmed, seeded, and cut into ¼-inch slices

Freshly ground black pepper

3 plum tomatoes, diced

¾ pound penne pasta plus ¼ pound for tomorrow's lunch (if desired)

½ cup thawed frozen peas

½ cup heavy cream

½ cup freshly grated Parmesan cheese

¼ cup fresh flat-leaf parsley leaves, finely chopped

At the shop:

½ cup freshly grated Parmesan cheese

¼ cup fresh flat-leaf parsley leaves, chopped

Salt

Freshly ground black pepper

Serve immediately, or let cool and transfer the dish to an airtight container. It will keep for 2 to 3 days in the refrigerator.

At the shop: Reheat the pasta. Serve with the cheese and parsley, and season as needed with salt and pepper.

Variation: You could easily make a lighter, vegetarian version by skipping the sausage and adding slightly parboiled broccoli or cauliflower instead. If you do, consider adding a pinch of hot pepper when you add the tomatoes.

A CZECH SENSE OF ECONOMY AND FOOD

Thirty years ago, the best restaurant in Seattle was Labuznik, run with an iron fist by Peter Cipra. He butchered his own meats (and, they would murmur, some of his staff). He saved every scrap from chopping vegetables and threw that into the stockpot, and he cooked every single dinner. He was a hard man, from a hard youth and a hard land; his only obvious soft spot was for children. Both of my children learned the taste of food from Peter Cipra.

The restaurant closed fifteen years ago, and Peter died in December 2011. As it is to many a restaurateur, lunch was important and private to him—a chance to use the wonderful ends and bits and sauces of the night before. No one closed his or her restaurant each night with more care and ferocity than Cipra. He saved food as if it were live, precious, and crucial. He had hundreds of storage containers and took particular care that whatever was to be saved had a proper container, with as little room for air as possible.

One busy holiday season, we asked him to make us a pasta that we could use for lunch. There would be six of us and not much time to prepare. He dropped by with this Penne Pasta with Sausage, Pepper, and Peas, in two plastic containers filled to the brim.

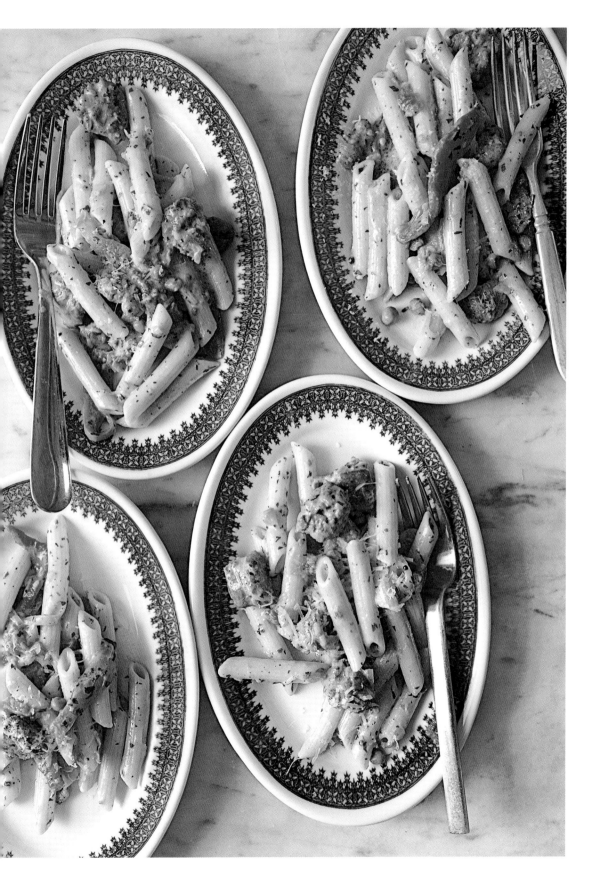

Lentil Soup, Pasta, and Beans, to Boot

SERVES FOUR.

At the shop:

1 cup lentil soup, or 1 can (12 ounces) creamy chicken soup

1 cup cooked pasta tossed with olive oil, Parmesan cheese, and salt (optional)

1 cup white bean soup or other bean soup (optional)

Salt

Freshly ground black pepper

½ cup freshly grated Parmesan cheese

1 tablespoon olive oil

2 tablespoons fresh flat-leaf parsley leaves, chopped

In truth, this recipe did not seem like a wonderful insight or grand possibility. We simply had most of the parts and added a few of the finishing details. But now it is one of our favorites.

You can either make the soups at home or purchase them. We buy the lentil soup from a wonderful Turkish café nearby; usually we buy enough for a couple of lunches. I had made too much pasta the night before, so I simply put some olive oil and Parmesan and salt on it and brought it in to add to a future lunch. And we had not quite finished a white bean soup.

I heated the pasta, added the lentils, and was about to serve it, when I remembered the white beans and tossed them in, as well. A little parsley and grated Parmesan, and it seemed a perfect fit.

You should have some extra plain, cooked pasta from Tuesday's lunch, which will come in handy. The bean soup is a grand addition, but do not worry if you do not have it. A trio is a wonder, but a duet is also fine.

At the shop: Heat the lentil soup, then reheat the pasta, if using, and add the bean soup, if using, adding a small splash of warmed water to them all. Then pour the warm lentil soup over the pasta. Fold the soups together, and heat again for a short time.

Taste and add salt, if needed, and certainly pepper. Add half the Parmesan and fold it into the soup. Serve the soup in warmed bowls, with a drizzle of oil, parsley, and the remaining Parmesan, all on the surface. If you can grill some bread, that is a perfect complement.

Variation: Instead of cheese, oil, and parsley, another fine option would be to top the soup with a dollop of Greek yogurt, cilantro, and lime juice, as shown here. Serve with lime.

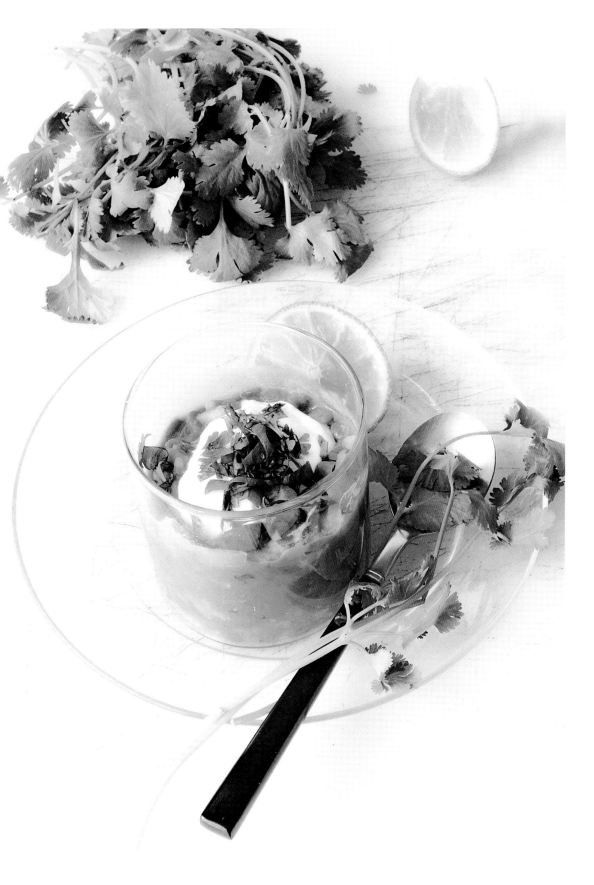

Poached Vegetables and Poached Salmon

SERVES FOUR.

This is a perfect spring dish, when the vegetables are all a bit smaller, the salmon are beginning their spring runs, and you are sick of winter fare. But, in truth, if you choose your vegetables carefully, you can make this year-round and re-create a little of spring. The dill is important—my daughter now lives in Stockholm, and I have learned to honor dill. Also, the poached vegetables and salmon, like a soup or a slow-cooked stew, seem to gather flavor when served the next day, making this dish perfect for a lunch.

It may look complicated, but it is not. Simplify, if that helps. The most important detail is that poached salmon is wonderful for lunch and easy to serve and seems much more elegant than the simple labor it entails.

At home: Wash all the vegetables and leave them wet in two bowls—potatoes, carrots, and celery in one; fava, asparagus, ramps or garlic, leeks, and peas in another.

In a wide saucepan, bring 2 cups of water and 1 cup of the white wine to a boil. Add 1 bay leaf, half of the onion, ½ cup of the oil, the juice of 1 lemon, and 1 teaspoon of the salt, and bring the liquid back to a rolling boil. Add one sprig of dill and the vegetables—potatoes first, then carrots and celery. Cook this first wave for 3 minutes, then add the second group to the mix—favas, asparagus, ramps, leeks, and peas—and cook for 3 minutes more.

Lift the vegetables out of the liquid immediately. You do not want them to sit in the poaching liquid and get soggy.

In a smaller pan, bring 2 cups of water and the remaining 1 cup of white wine to a boil. Add the remaining bay leaf, onion, oil, juice of 1 lemon, and 1 teaspoon salt, and return the mixture to a boil. Gently lay the salmon into the poaching liquid, add a whole sprig of the all-important dill, and let the liquid boil over the salmon. If your fillet is from the tail, it is thinner and may only need to poach for 5 minutes. If it is a center-cut piece, or thicker, it may need up to 8 minutes. You can see that the salmon is done by the color rising in the flesh (see the cut end) but also by touch, for it will have firmed.

Remove the pan from the heat, and let the salmon cool in the liquid (unlike the vegetables!). Store it in an airtight container, with ½ cup of its poaching liquid, and refrigerate.

At the shop: Bring the vegetables and the salmon out of the fridge

---

At home:

4 small new red potatoes, halved

8 small carrots, green tops still attached and trimmed to 1 inch

1 celery stalk, cut diagonally into 2-inch pieces

½ cup peeled fava beans, if available

8 to 10 thin asparagus spears, trimmed

2 ramps, if available, trimmed, or 1 clove garlic, minced

2 small leeks or spring onions, trimmed

½ cup fresh or thawed frozen peas

2 cups white wine

2 bay leaves

1 onion, halved

1 cup olive oil

2 lemons

2 teaspoons sea salt

2 sprigs fresh dill

1 pound wild salmon fillet, skinned, or 2 wild salmon steaks (½ pound each), skinned

At the shop:

2 sprigs fresh dill

12 cornichons

1 tablespoon mayonnaise

Salt

Freshly ground black pepper

10 minutes before serving, so the sharpest cold is off them. Add a whole sprig of the dill on top, a couple of cornichons on the side, and a dollop of mayonnaise, with some extra chopped dill and a couple of finely chopped cornichons mixed into the mayonnaise. At the very last, add a little salt and 2 grinds of black pepper.

A FRENCH DUDE AND SPRING DISTINCTIONS

I was in Montana last spring with Philippe, a French winemaker. We were party to a wonderful anniversary celebration with twenty-one people, on a tour from Missoula to Butte to Wise River, eating all the way. Philippe was fascinated by Montana, for it is particular in very particular ways and has a very complicated history with the American Indian, and all of that has a great allure to a Frenchman. He noticed the brilliance of the knife shops, and the freshness of the eggs, and the taste of the water, and the ample cut of the beef.

It was Philippe who spotted the garlic at the Saturday Market in Missoula. "Look," he said. "It is perfectly formed, not too grand. The skin comes off completely, and the taste is clear, not dull, and not bitter. It must be the cold nights. It is the best garlic in America," he declared.

"Do you know what I am, here in Montana?" Philippe announced one morning at breakfast. "I am the French Dude!" He was honored to have the title, having overheard the waitresses talking about his order for eggs.

Later that day, after dinner, I brought out some French cheeses as a final detail for the celebration. I showed them to Philippe, and he was quite pleased. "But," he said, "you must put the soft ones in the microwave—only for eight to ten seconds, not more." He was right; it made all the difference.

It is always a good sign when details carry many times their weight. For me, it is easier to cook well when I am aware that they do, indeed, make all the difference.

Couscous with Roasted Cherry Tomatoes, Green Onions, Feta, Parsley, and Mint

SERVES FOUR.

At home:

½ pound cherry tomatoes

Salt

Freshly ground black pepper

I cup couscous

6 scallions, roughly chopped

½ cup fresh mint leaves, chopped

½ cup fresh flat-leaf parsley leaves, chopped

I lemon

¼ cup olive oil

½ cup crumbled feta cheese

At the shop:

¼ cup fresh flat-leaf parsley leaves, chopped

¼ cup fresh mint leaves, chopped

I cup Greek yogurt

6 pita breads, grilled or slightly heated in microwave (optional)

This dish improves by sitting in the refrigerator for a few hours or overnight; the flavors begin to mingle and share. But take the chill off it before serving, and at the very last, add some fresh parsley and mint, to bring it completely into the present tense.

There is a wonderful lightness to couscous. And that makes the parsley and mint seem even more important. It is a wonderful dish in the summer. But it is fine in the winter, when the colors and the taste of a couscous seem a signal from warmer lands.

Also, this recipe is a good catchall for the end of the week. Should you have any leftovers, a bit of salmon or sausage or chicken or lentils, mix each in a separate bowl with some of the couscous, add a little lemon juice and parsley, taste, and serve. Keep each one specific—to the lentils, for example, you might also add a little yogurt, to the salmon, add a little avocado. With pita bread, or any soft French bread, you can concoct small servings of each.

At home: Preheat the oven to 350°F. Oil a shallow roasting pan.

Lay the tomatoes, cut-side up, in a tight bunch in the prepared pan. Salt and pepper them. Roast for 30 minutes, then remove from the oven and let cool.

Meanwhile, bring a cup of water to a boil in a small pan. Set a large bowl on the warmed stove top for a few moments. Place the couscous in the warm bowl, add salt and pepper, then pour in ¾ cup boiling water. Cover the bowl well with plastic. Fluff the couscous with a fork every 5 minutes or so, re-covering it after each time, and let cool.

To assemble the dish, first add the scallions, nearly all the mint and parsley (save a little for the very last), the juice of the lemon, and the oil. Fold it all together, but only with 3 or 4 turns—you are not trying to mash it. Then add the tomatoes; they will be a little fragile, so be careful. Add the feta, and give the mixture a turn. Taste and adjust the seasoning. Finish with the rest of the mint and parsley, and even try to get a few last drops out of the squeezed lemon. Taste for salt and pepper.

Transfer the couscous to an airtight container and refrigerate it. It must take on its own smells and liquids, no others.

At the shop: Serve the couscous with the parsley and mint, yogurt, and warm pita breads.

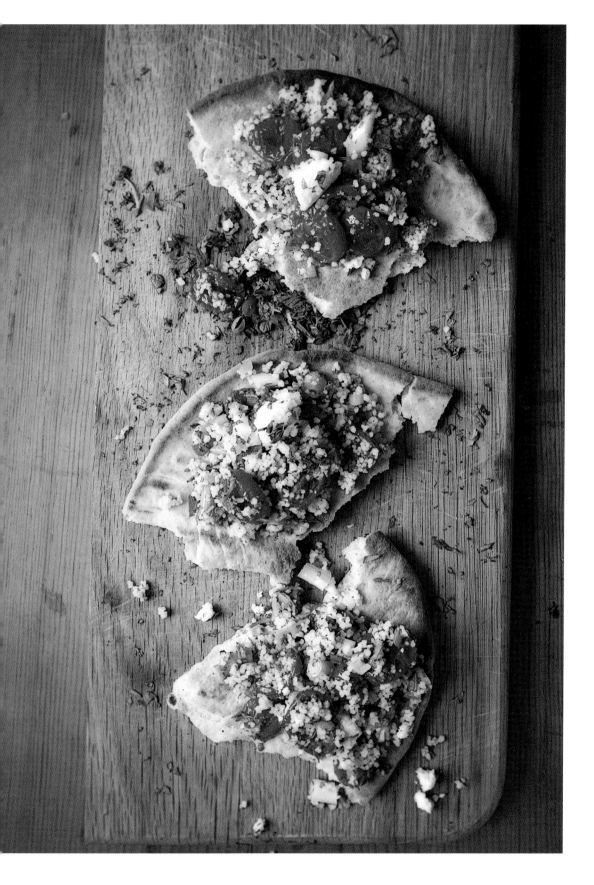

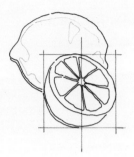

WEEK 2

In the second week of lunches, the meatballs carry their weight, but so do the lentils and the white beans. Again, you have a little prep to do at home, even a Sunday chore of making meatballs. At the shop, you should have the olive oil, vinegar, Parmesan, and parsley from the previous week, but check your supply of these. Get some bread for sandwiches, some butter, fresh lemons, lots of arugula, a red onion, and more yogurt. On Tuesday night, you will want to make a quick batch of green sauce to bring in the next day. By Friday, you will need pita bread or white corn tortillas. With luck, you have some green sauce left from the bean soup—if not, buy some salsa when you are picking up the pita or tortillas.

There are a couple herbs that would be perfect for the week—basil for the meatballs and thyme for the tuna. If you can find them, wonderful—they will also help with the Friday cleanup—but the dishes are fine without them.

Meatballs for Later

———————

MAKES ABOUT 24 MEATBALLS.

I suppose everyone knows how to make meatballs, though no one seems to actually make them. Here is a refresher recipe. I love the fact that different towns in France compete each year for the national best-meatball award—there must be something to the different recipes if you can make a contest of it!

They are, of course, quite easy to make; they simply need a little attention in the making. If you make them on a Sunday and they make it to work, you can easily turn them into any number of lunches, including the two on pages 146 and 150.

For the beef, do not choose the extra lean; you need a little fat for meatballs. And try to get it from a butcher. It may seem silly to be picky about hamburger, but a supermarket's meat grinder can grind anything, of any age, and it will still look like hamburger.

At home: Cut off all the crust from the bread, and cut the bread into slices. Reserve 2 slices, and cut the rest into ½-inch cubes.

Heat the milk or cream in a small saucepan until it is hot but not boiling, and add the reserved 2 slices bread. Mash the bread a little until it absorbs the milk and the milk starts to dissolve the bread into a mush. Remove from the heat and let cool.

Place the bread cubes in the bowl of a food processor and pulse for 1 minute or until the cubes are broken down into crumbs. You will need about 2 loose cups of bread crumbs. Lay them out in an even layer on a rimmed baking sheet, and place them in the oven. Set the oven to 400°F. Watch the crumbs; they will need to toast for 8 to 10 minutes, just until brown. Remove the pan from the oven, and set aside to cool. Leave the oven on.

Once the crumbs are cool, toss them back into the food processor, and pulse to grind them finer. Alternatively, place them in a large zip-top bag and crush them with a rolling pin. Pour the bread crumbs back onto the rimmed baking sheet and set aside.

Crack the egg into a small bowl and whisk until smooth. Mix in the Parmesan, parsley, nutmeg, ¼ cup of the oil, and the rosemary, sage, and thyme. Set aside.

Heat a 10-inch sauté pan over medium heat for a moment, and then add the remaining 2 tablespoons oil and the onions. Cook for 5 minutes, until the onions soften, then add the carrots and cook, stirring, for 2 minutes. Add the garlic and stir again. Sauté for 2 to 3 minutes;

At home:

1 loaf day-old country white bread

¼ cup milk or cream

1 egg, at room temperature

½ cup freshly grated Parmesan cheese

½ cup fresh flat-leaf parsley leaves, chopped

1 teaspoon freshly grated nutmeg

¼ cup + 2 tablespoons olive oil

1 teaspoon fresh rosemary, chopped

1 teaspoon fresh sage, chopped

1 teaspoon fresh thyme leaves, chopped

1 onion, finely chopped

2 carrots, finely chopped

2 garlic cloves, finely chopped

Salt

Freshly ground black pepper

1½ pounds ground beef or 1 pound ground beef and ½ pound ground pork or veal

do not let it burn—either shake the pan or stir well. Season with salt and pepper, then remove from the heat and set aside to cool.

Wash your hands well. Put the meat in a large bowl, season well with salt and pepper, and, with your hands, mix it together for a minute or two. Make a well in the center of the meat and add the bread mush. Scrape the onion mixture into the bowl over the bread mush. Mix all this for a minute and then add the egg mixture and fold it all together. You are simply folding the meat, for no more than another minute.

When everything seems to be evenly distributed, wash your hands again and leave them wet. Scoop a heaping tablespoon of the mixture and roll it in your palms until it is round. Lay the meatball on top of the bread crumbs and repeat with the remaining meat. Keep them about 2 inches in diameter, and of the same size, so they will cook evenly. Only roll them in your palm for 10 seconds or so, just enough to shape them.

When all the meatballs have been formed, roll them around a little to cover their surface with the bread crumbs. Pour a little oil into a roasting pan, and place the breaded meatballs in the pan. Roast the meatballs for 25 minutes—if you can, open the oven after 10 minutes and turn them; it will keep them from getting too flat on one side.

Remove the pan from the oven, taste a meatball, and add salt and pepper as needed. Transfer the meatballs to a wire rack above some paper towels and let them cool. Or you could add them to a tomato sauce that you have started—they are ready to go. (I love having tomato sauce on hand, but it seems even more obvious when I am making meatballs.) The meatballs will keep in an airtight container in the refrigerator for up to a week.

————————————

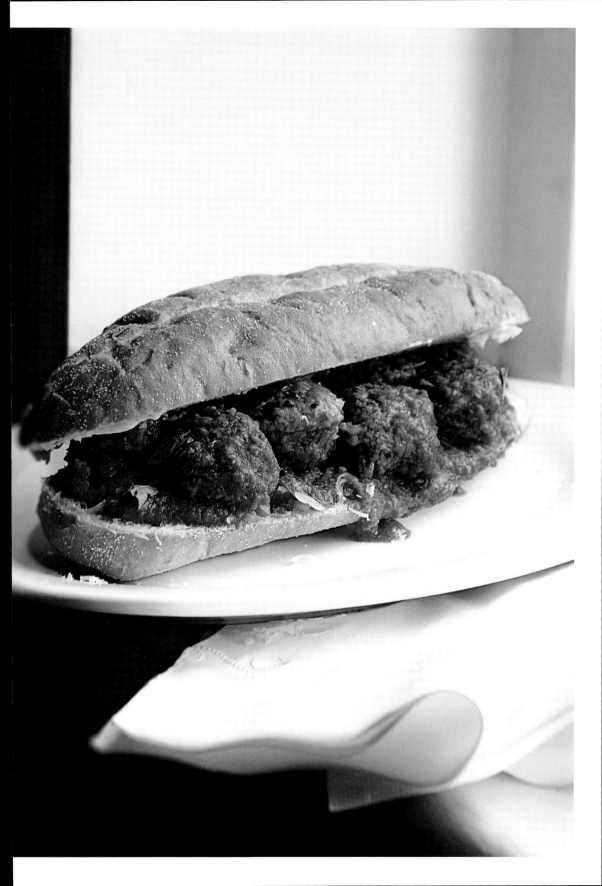

Meatball Sandwich

————————

SERVES FOUR.

Very straightforward, this. The only trick is to get the sauce and the meatballs hot enough to melt the butter and soften the Parmesan. Pick up the rolls on your way to work, and make sure they are fresh. If you buy extra, they will come in handy again on Wednesday. The basil is only truly essential for this if the sauce is somewhat bland.

At the shop: Heat the meatballs and sauce together and then taste the sauce—it may need salt and considerable pepper.

Cut the bread or rolls crosswise so that they open like a book, with one side still attached. Butter the inside well, using all of the butter, then add the meatballs and sauce and quickly top with the Parmesan. Then add some basil, if using, and 2 grinds of black pepper, and serve.

It should be a little messy, both to look at and to eat. Serve it with marinated vegetables to the side, such as cauliflower and red onions and red peppers—sweet and sour tastes that can compete with the mess.

————————

At the shop:

12 meatballs (see page 143)

½ cup homemade or store-bought tomato sauce

Salt

Freshly ground black pepper

4 ciabatta rolls, pieces of French bread, or hoagie rolls (anything soft inside and not hard-crusted)

4 tablespoons butter

½ cup freshly grated Parmesan cheese

6 basil leaves, cut or torn into shreds (optional)

Lentils with Asparagus, Arugula, and Parmesan

SERVES FOUR.

This is a lovely dish, but it is at its best if constructed just before serving. It is the asparagus you must be careful with—if soaked or cooked even moments too long, it loses its place.

This is also a good dish for experimenting with different lentils, from the very small black beluga to the larger lenticchie verdi.

Also, don't forget to boil extra rice when making this recipe and to save it for Wednesday's lunch; it can be employed again on Friday, so don't skimp. Buy plenty of arugula, too, which comes in handy again on Thursday and Friday.

At home: Rinse the lentils well. Bring a pot of water to a boil, with a piece of garlic in it, add the lentils, and cook for 15 to 20 minutes, until they are soft. Drain and rinse the lentils, and place them in a bowl. Add salt and the cooked rice and mix to combine. Taste and season with salt and pepper, as needed, then add 1 tablespoon of the vinaigrette.

Trim the asparagus and soak it in cold water for 3 to 4 minutes (no more, or it will waterlog the asparagus). Bring a saucepan or sauté pan of salted water, enough to cover the asparagus, to a boil, and cook the asparagus. If the asparagus is fresh and thin, it may take only a minute. If it is thick, it may take 3 minutes. If it is from thousands of miles away, check it with a thin knife after 4 minutes.

Drain the asparagus and cut it into 2-inch pieces while still hot. Put them in a small bowl, then add salt and the remaining 1 tablespoon of vinaigrette, and give it all a very quick toss. Store the cooked asparagus and vinaigrette in airtight containers.

At the shop: Bring the rice and lentils and asparagus to room temperature.

Chop ½ of the arugula and fold that into the lentils and rice. Combine 2 tablespoons of the Parmesan and half of the cooked asparagus, and fold into the lentils and rice. Lightly portion out the mixture among 4 plates, and divide the remaining asparagus among the plates, laying it on top. Top with the remaining arugula, vinaigrette, and Parmesan. The dish must reflect the different layers and textures and weights of its components.

At home:

1 cup lentils

1 garlic clove

Salt

½ cup cooked Carnaroli rice or any long-grain rice, plus ½ cup for tomorrow's lunch (if desired)

Freshly ground black pepper

2 tablespoons A Very Good Basic Vinaigrette (see page 51)

½ pound fresh asparagus

At the shop:

2 cups arugula

½ cup freshly grated Parmesan cheese

2 tablespoons A Very Good Basic Vinaigrette (see page 51)

Variation: Instead of asparagus, try this dish with cauliflower, especially in the winter. Break the cauliflower into medium florets, and cook them in a pan of boiling, unsalted water for about 15 minutes. You want the cauliflower slightly underdone, not mushy. When the cauliflower is nearly done, throw ½ cup golden raisins into the pan with the florets, then drain. Incorporate the cauliflower and raisins as you would the asparagus.

PAVAROTTI AT THE SHOP

Some good soul had the sense to videotape the famous tenor Luciano Pavarotti making lunch in a studio the day after Thanksgiving. Pavarotti was obviously thrilled with the prospect, for he had a broad table of leftover ingredients and could hardly contain his enthusiasm for how wonderfully they could be combined.

Into the sauté pan went some stuffing, a bit of chopped garlic, pieces of turkey, turnips, small white onions, carrots, and brussels sprouts. Pavarotti thinned the gravy with cream, stock, and wine and added that to a well he'd made in the center of the pan. Then more garlic and parsley. He cracked pepper over it all, tossing well. The linguine had been cooking at the back of the stove; he tasted it for doneness, pulled the pot's colander up, laid the pasta, still dripping wet, in the center of the pan, and then gave the pan a great shake to mix it all.

Laughing, Pavarotti held a chunk of Parmesan above it all and grated it in every direction—a toss, another grating, and it was done. A great Italian tenor, with everything at hand, who enjoyed the pleasure of food, the pleasure of company, and the pleasure of a lunch assembled from many parts.

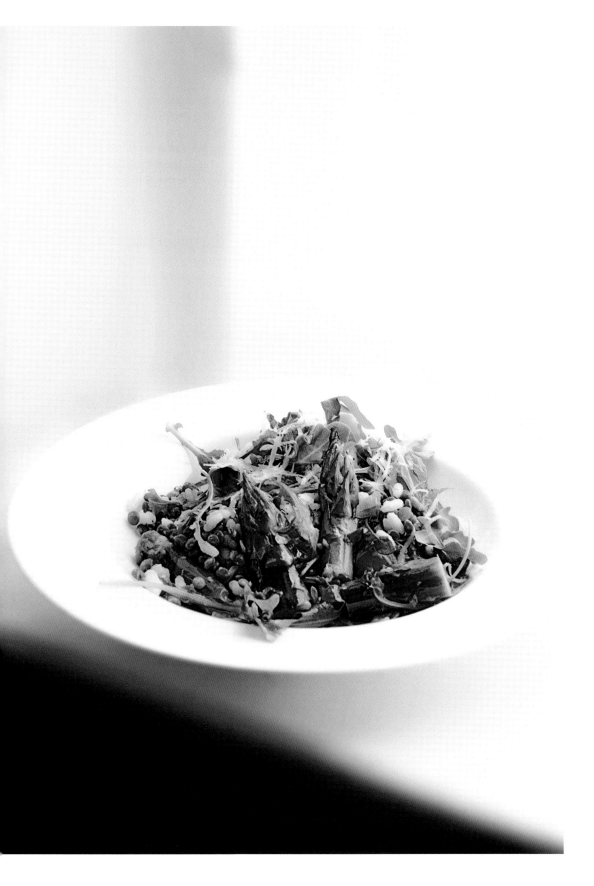

Bean Soup and Meatballs

SERVES FOUR.

At the shop:

12 meatballs (see page 143)

½ cup cooked rice

2 cups white bean soup or lentil soup (see pages 61 and 74)

½ cup Green Sauce (see page 35) or pesto

½ lemon

4 pieces bread

¼ cup olive oil

1 avocado (optional)

Meatballs love company. This dish is best with smooth cannellini bean soup, which can either be purchased from a nearby shop or made at home, and should you have any leftovers from the Lentils with Asparagus, Arugula, and Parmesan (see page 147), add them, as well. Simply fold them in after you have heated the soup, check for seasoning and temperature, and then add the meatballs. You will get a sense of how generous a white bean soup can be—it works perfectly on its own but is also a fine base for other things.

It does not sound like much, but if the soup is delicate and smooth, the meatballs good, and the green sauce a little tart, then this is a very delicious lunch, especially served with something that combines crunchy and smooth.

At the shop: Reheat the meatballs; be certain they are heated through.

Combine the rice with the soup, and heat it until almost too hot to eat. Divide it among 4 bowls, and fold in 3 meatballs per bowl. You can cut the meatballs into smaller pieces or in half if the proportion seems better.

Top each bowl with a good spoonful (about 2 tablespoons) of the green sauce and a squeeze of lemon juice.

Toast or grill the bread (slightly stale bread left over from Monday will do the trick) and serve it alongside, sprinkled with oil. Or better yet, cut it into strips, drizzle it with oil, sprinkle salt and pepper on it, and top with a slice of avocado, if using.

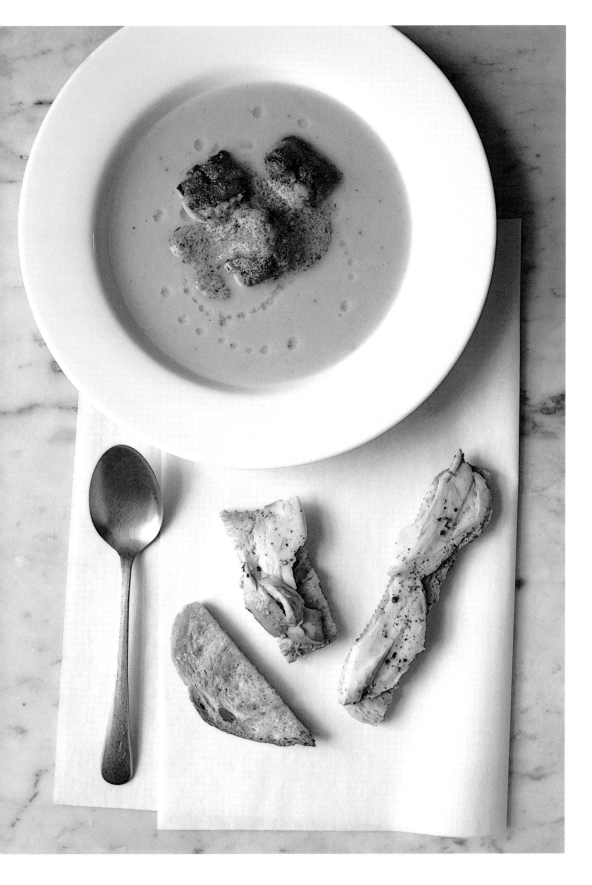

A Salad of Tuna, Beans, and Red Onion

SERVES FOUR.

Once prepped, this is an easily assembled lunch. It has two lives, in a sense: There is its freshness, when first made, and then there is its taste after marinating. They are slightly different but both good.

At home: Cut the tuna into 8 to 10 square pieces. Put them into a stainless-steel bowl, and toss with a drizzle of the oil. Coat the pieces and then add the cracked pepper and a good pinch of salt. Toss well to coat them all.

Heat the remaining oil in a sauté pan until the oil shimmers. It must be hot enough to sear the tuna. Add the tuna pieces and turn them every 30 seconds; they are only going to be in the heat for 3 minutes total. Lift the tuna pieces out of the pan and set them aside to cool on paper towels. Once cool, store them in an airtight container in the refrigerator.

At the shop: Take the tuna out of the fridge, and drain the cooked cannellini beans in a colander.

Put the onion rings into a small stainless-steel bowl. Add cold water to cover and let sit for 15 minutes—it will sweeten the onion. Just before tossing the salad, lift out the onion, squeeze the rings in a paper towel, and set them aside to dry.

This is a salad best kept loose-limbed, so pick your biggest bowl to do the mixing. Place the arugula, a pinch of salt, and all the dressing in the bowl, and toss very quickly. Add the onions and toss. Add the beans and toss a bit more. This is a good place to add another pinch of salt. Quickly, and lightly, divide the salad among 4 plates.

The tuna must then go into the salad bowl, to catch a little of what dressing is left—it is not there to soak, only to quickly pass through. Lift the pieces out and lay them over the greens on each plate, dividing the pieces equally. Pluck off the leaves from the sprig of thyme, sprinkle the leaves on top, and add a final grind of pepper.

Should you have any leftovers, store them in the airtight container, and serve them alongside a sandwich later on, or as part of the end-of-the-week cleanup the next day. Crack some black pepper over the top, and add a squirt of lemon just before serving.

At home:

8 ounces fresh tuna fillet

½ cup olive oil

2 tablespoons freshly cracked black pepper (not ground)

Sea salt

At the shop:

1 cup cannellini beans, soaked, cooked, and stored in their liquid (see page 59)

1 red onion, thinly sliced

2 cups arugula

Salt

¼ cup salad dressing (see A Salad with Plenty of Parts, page 53)

1 sprig fresh thyme

Freshly ground black pepper

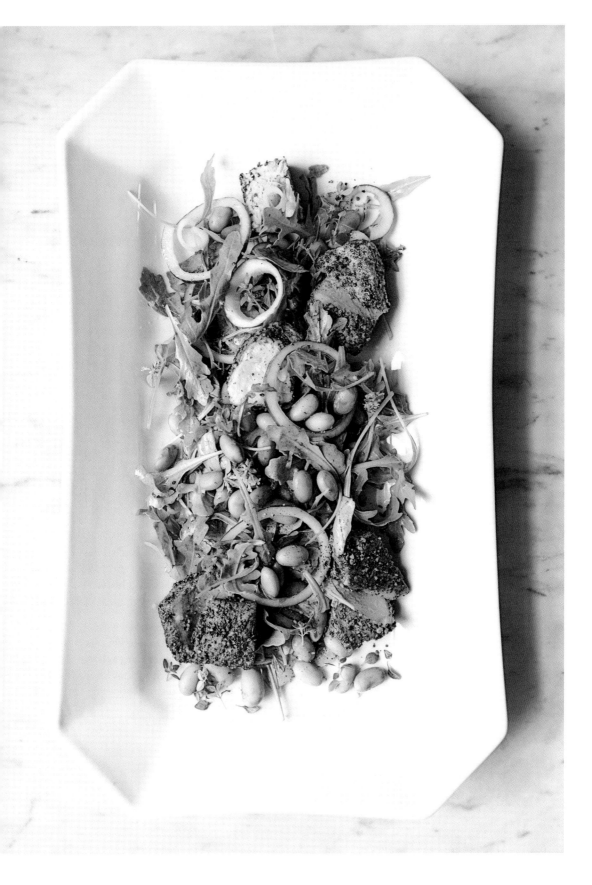

End-of-the-Week Cleanup

If you have made lunches all week, then you have some decisions to make by Friday—food that needs to be served, green sauce that will not last through the weekend, half a container of yogurt from the previous Friday. You have to clean up the week. There are no recipes for this; it is simply the pleasure of putting parts together.

We use white corn tortillas to make the cleanup easier and fun. They are available in most grocery stores, but you may find places selling freshly made tortillas in your neighborhood.

Use your microwave or panini press to heat them. Lay out the food you need to use, in its bowls or containers, so you can clearly see it. And choose your largest serving tray or platter to be your stage. Make certain that any food you want to use comes out of its container—it never looks as good crammed into a corner. Sprinkle some with parsley, add a little oil, and make all your leftovers look their very best.

In smaller bowls, make a presentation of a little mustard, some chutney, some pickles, olives, yogurt, hummus, salsa—whatever you have.

In slightly larger bowls, spoon the leftover beans, the not-quite-finished rice, or the lentils.

Clean and dry any lettuces or greens, and lay them on a plate. Trim the leftover half avocado and slice it thinly and squirt lemon juice on it so it does not brown. Do the same with the leftover half apple or pear.

Now put a few things together. On a few tortillas, spread some salsa and some chopped lettuce. Spoon a little rice over the lettuce, and lay some avocado on it, with a squirt of lemon and a sprinkle of salt. Or put lentils on the pita with a little yogurt and some mint. Fold and serve. You are now an open-air market of your own. Lunch at the shop—it is your bazaar.

You might even invite some guests; it is a tribute to what you have done all week. When the Friday lunch is over, you should have a good handful of clean storage containers awaiting new assignments, some space in the refrigerator, and some pleasure in that the meals were a success.

TO FINISH

Lunch is not a full orchestra. It is a half-hour rehearsal, with but a handful of instruments. You are never precisely certain who will show up, or what you will play.

But you have what you need: good oil and vinegar, a lemon, a piece of cheese, sea salt, and black pepper.

A few greens, some firm olives, butter, and fresh bread. A handful of rice, some lovely white beans, a bit of pasta. Lucky you.

FANCY KITCHENS, LOVELY LUNCH

I remember my first lunch at a shop. I went with my friend, Bill Stout, the remarkable San Francisco bookseller and architect, to the Boffi kitchen showroom in Milan to work on the details for a house in California. It was a very long morning of checking and reworking details of every sort—a Boffi kitchen is an elegant and complicated affair.

At half past noon, the wonderful and extraordinarily patient Boffi director stopped and laid her drafting pencil at the table edge. She went to the large front showroom windows that looked out over the bustle of Milan and pulled the shades down three-quarters of the way. She and an assistant prepared lunch for the four of us in the back room—fresh bread, tomato, basil, and mozzarella sandwiches, a small glass of very cold white wine, and a salad of white cannellini beans, olive oil, and arugula. We talked and told stories and, for the moment, were very far from the difficult complications of our work.

Each of us had a bottle of water, and each of us sipped a very tiny espresso to finish. Then a thimbleful of Scotch. Everyone laughed, up went the shades, and we were back at work. I decided then that I would shut my bookshop at half past noon each workday, pull down the shades, and have lunch. I would consider it a great honor, and a great lesson.

CONVERSION CHARTS

WEIGHT EQUIVALENTS: The metric weights given in this chart are not exact equivalents, but have been rounded up or down slightly to make measuring easier.

VOLUME EQUIVALENTS: These are not exact equivalents for American cups and spoons, but have been rounded up or down slightly to make measuring easier.

AVOIRDUPOIS	METRIC
¼ oz	7 g
½ oz	15 g
1 oz	30 g
2 oz	55 g
3 oz	85 g
4 oz	115 g
5 oz	140 g
6 oz	170 g
7 oz	200 g
8 oz (½ lb)	225 g
9 oz	255 g
10 oz	280 g
11 oz	310 g
12 oz	340 g
13 oz	370 g
14 oz	400 g
15 oz	430 g
16 oz (1 lb)	455 g
1½ lb	680 g
2 lb	910 g
2½ lb	1.2 kg
3 lb	1.4 kg
4 lb	1.8 kg

AMERICAN	METRIC	IMPERIAL
¼ tsp	1.2 ml	
½ tsp	2.5 ml	
1 tsp	5.0 ml	
½ Tbsp (1.5 tsp)	7.5 ml	
1 Tbsp (3 tsp)	15 ml	
¼ cup (4 Tbsp)	60 ml	2 fl oz
⅓ cup (5 Tbsp)	75 ml	2.5 fl oz
½ cup (8 Tbsp)	120 ml	4 fl oz
⅔ cup (10 Tbsp)	165 ml	5.5 fl oz
¾ cup (12 Tbsp)	175 ml	6 fl oz
1 cup (16 Tbsp)	240 ml	8 fl oz
1¼ cups	300 ml	10 fl oz (½ pint)
1½ cups	350 ml	12 fl oz
2 cups (1 pint)	480 ml	16 fl oz
2½ cups	600 ml	20 fl oz (1 pint)
1 quart	1 liter	32 fl oz

OVEN MARK	F	C	GAS
Very cool	250–275	120–135	½–1
Cool	300	150	2
Warm	325	165	3
Moderate	350	175	4
Moderately hot	375	190	5
	400	205	6
Hot	425	220	7
	450	230	8
Very hot	475	250	9

ACKNOWLEDGMENTS

It is an honor and a task to have a book published, and it takes a remarkable ship of people to get it published:

to all the people I have met who love to cook and love to share their cooking.

to Michael Jacobs, the president and CEO of ABRAMS, who said quite simply, "Let's do the Lunch book," and then said, "I will find you an editor who gets it."

to Laura Dozier, my editor, who has always loved this book, even when it was but an awkward and unwashed youth.

to Les Canalistes, Melissa Hamilton and Christopher Hirsheimer, who said yes at every moment and who took every picture. They knew more than I knew even to ask.

to my quite remarkable staff, all of them over all the thirty-five years, for they knew it was never a typical job but often a very good lunch.

to the many people who have supported the shop—their loyalty and friend-ship are literally all of the difference.

to my daughter, Nina, and my son, Joe, who love to go out and love to come home—it is always a simple honor to cook for them.

And to my wife, Colleen, who was a little jealous that a book could so bra-zenly gobble up and chew on such chunks of time. Her illustrations are the quiet grace of the book, as I knew they would be.

INDEX

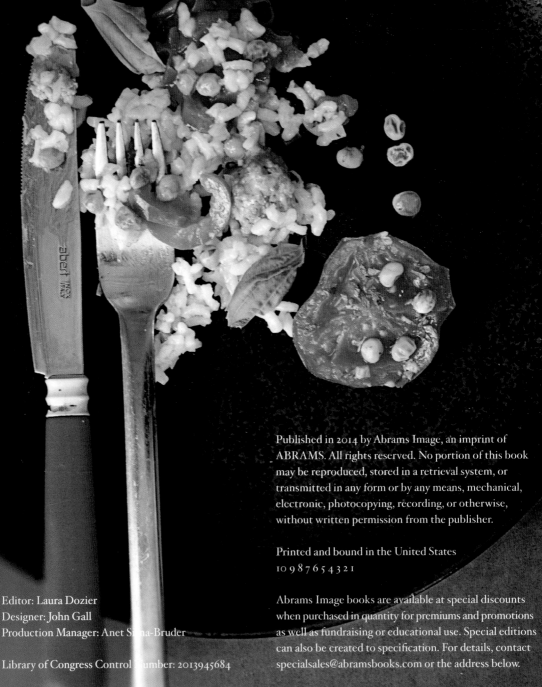

Published in 2014 by Abrams Image, an imprint of
ABRAMS. All rights reserved. No portion of this book
may be reproduced, stored in a retrieval system, or
transmitted in any form or by any means, mechanical,
electronic, photocopying, recording, or otherwise,
without written permission from the publisher.

Printed and bound in the United States
10 9 8 7 6 5 4 3 2 1

Editor: Laura Dozier
Designer: John Gall
Production Manager: Anet Sirna-Bruder

Library of Congress Control Number: 2013945684

ISBN: 978-1-4197-1065-0

Text copyright © 2014 Peter Miller
Photographs copyright © 2014
Christopher Hirsheimer and Melissa Hamilton
Illustrations copyright © 2014 Colleen Miller

ABRAMS
THE ART OF BOOKS SINCE 1949

115 West 18th Street
New York, NY 10011
www.abramsbooks.com